MEDICAL MAVERICKS
VOLUME ONE

HUGH DESAIX RIORDAN, M.D.

Bio-Communications Press
3100 North Hillside
Wichita, Kansas 67219 USA

MEDICAL MAVERICKS
Volume I

Copyright © 1988
This book may not be reproduced in whole or in part, by mimeograph or any other means, without permission. For information address:

BIO-COMMUNICATIONS PRESS
3100 North Hillside Avenue
Wichita, Kansas 67219 USA

ISBN 0-942333-07-1
Library of Congress Catalog Card Number: 88-63321

First Edition

Published in The United States of America

cover drawing by Moore Anderson

BCP and Bio-Communications Press are service marks of
The Olive W. Garvey Center
for the Improvement of Human Functioning, Inc.

"If the science of medicine is not to be lowered to the rank of a mere mechanical profession, it must pre-occupy itself with its history…"

EMILE LITTRÉ

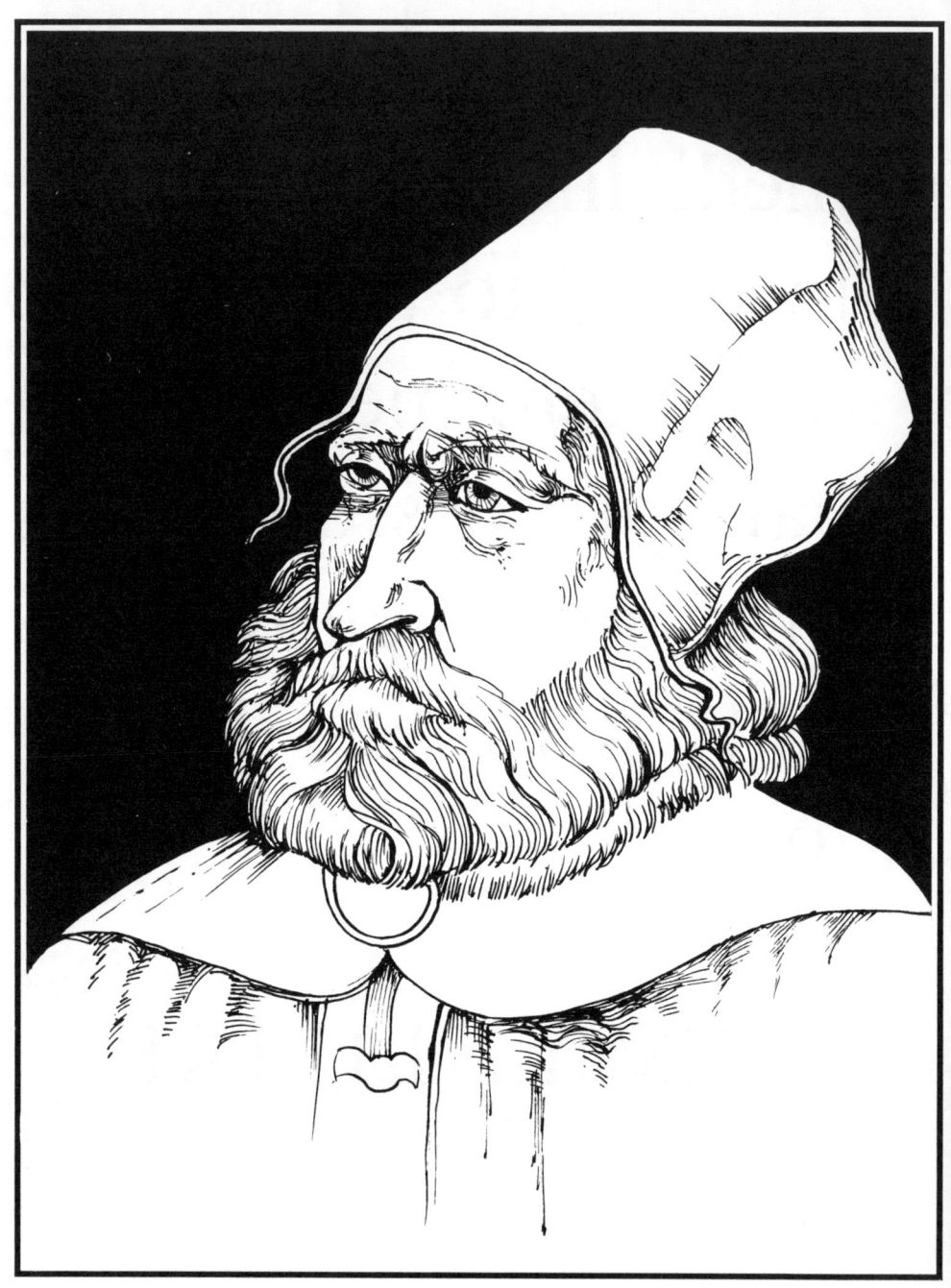

GALEN

TABLE OF CONTENTS

MAVERICK	vi
DEDICATION	vii
ACKNOWLEDGEMENTS	viii
FOREWORD	ix
LEOPOLD AUENBRUGGER	1
ROGER BACON	5
ELIZABETH BLACKWELL	9
ZABDIEL BOYLSTON	15
PIETRO D'ABANO	21
CLAUDIUS GALENUS	25
JOSEPH GOLDBERGER	31
GEORG GRODDECK	37
WILLIAM HARVEY	43
HENRY HILL HICKMAN	47
HIPPOCRATES	49
ANTOINE LAVOISIER	55
JOSEPH LISTER	59
EPHRAIM MCDOWELL	65
WILLIAM MORTON	71
PARACELSUS	79
LOUIS PASTEUR	83
MIGUEL SERVETO OR SERVETUS	87
POSTSCRIPT	89
CHRONOLOGICAL LIST	90
FOOTNOTES	91
BIBLIOGRAPHY	97

MAVERICK

The word maverick is derived from an American pioneer, Samuel A. Maverick, who chose to not brand his cattle. Through usage the word maverick, in addition to meaning an unbranded range animal, has come to mean an independent individual who refuses to conform to his group.

This book is about such independent individuals who followed the advice found in this anonymous quotation.

> *Do not follow where*
> *The path may lead*
> *Go instead where*
> *There is no path*
> *And leave a trail*

DEDICATION

This book is dedicated to the memory of all those medical doctors who, since history has been recorded, have contributed to the progress of the science and art of medicine.

This book is also dedicated to the countless numbers of those people we call patients who have, through the ages, endured much, suffered greatly and benefitted considerably from those who have practiced the science and art of medicine.

This book is dedicated to the maverick in you—that wonderful element perhaps obvious, perhaps hidden which moved you to choose to read this bit of writing.

And lastly, this book is dedicated to my wonderful, loving family—Jan, Michael, Neil, Teresa, Renee, Brian and Quinn—each of whom has a touch of the maverick spirit.

H.D.R.

ACKNOWLEDGEMENTS

The initial draft of this book was initiated several years ago. This first volume of a planned trilogy has come to fruition following arduous research, dedicated input and skillful editing by Jeanne Johnston and Rebecca Burke.

The final production of this volume has been made possible by the fine efforts of Barbara Nichols of Bio-Communications Press, Teresa Riordan who performed final editing and Moore Anderson whose sketch of Galen appears on the cover. I am most grateful to each of you.

The recent impetus for actually getting this book to press came from many positive comments made by physicians who heard individual excerpts of *Medical Mavericks* on my radio series "Just for the Health of It."

Many thanks to you medical doctors who said "I want to hear more."

H. D. R.

FOREWORD

Those who are superb chronological thinkers may prefer that the vignettes in this book were sequenced according to life span rather than alphabetically. For you, they are so listed on page 90.

Although there is considerable merit in using the chronologic approach, I, being something of a maverick myself, preferred not to follow that convention.

I did this in part because the underlying messages we receive from this material are timeless. Whether it is the most ancient Hippocrates or the more recent Goldberger the vignettes repeatedly reflect the wisdom of Schopenhauer's observation that new thought and new truths most often go through three stages. First they are ridiculed. Next they are violently opposed. Then, finally they are accepted as being self-evident.

H. D. R.

AUENBRUGGER

"I foresee very well that I shall encounter no little opposition to my views... I realize, however, that envy and blame and even hatred and calumny have never failed discoveries or have added to their perfection."[1]

Leopold Auenbrugger

Leopold Auenbrugger (1722-1809), born in Gratz, Austria, was the son of a prosperous innkeeper. His father taught him as a young boy how to judge the amount of wine in the casks by thumping them. Auenbrugger never forgot this lesson. With it as his basis, he later invented a new method of physical diagnosis using percussion to discover the presence and amount of fluid in the chest.

After receiving his medical degree, Auenbrugger was appointed physician to a Vienna hospital, the Spanish Military Hospital. He was bothered by the fact that many patients died of unknown diseases which were later discovered to be ailments of the chest. He was certain that pneumonia, tuberculosis, and other diseases could be recognized while the patients were still alive. He remembered how he had thumped the winecasks to find out how much wine remained in each and was convinced that the same principle could apply to the diagnosis of his patients' chest diseases.

He immediately started his investigation. He was often able to correlate his percussive findings with conditions found at the autopsy. He was also able to prove the existence of fluid by withdrawing fluid from his patients' lungs with a trocar. Soon he could distinguish immediately a healthy chest from a diseased chest.

After seven years of research, Auenbrugger felt that he had satisfactorily proven the value of his new diagnostic method. He published a ninety-five page booklet entitled *Inventum Novum* (1761), or *The New Invention That Enables the Physician from the Percussion of the Human Thorax to Detect the Diseases Hidden within the Chest.* In this booklet, Auenbrugger clearly described the method of percussion and mapped the sounds of the healthy or diseased chest when thumped in various places.

The book received scant attention, however. Many doctors absolutely ignored Auenbrugger's discovery. Auenbrugger was most distressed by the silence of a former professor of his, whom he greatly respected, Baron Van Swieten. Van Swieten, as well as another distinguished doctor, wrote a treatise on diseases of the chest a few years after the publication of *Inventum Novum*. But neither treatise mentions percussion and its possible value. Other physicians claimed that Auenbrugger was merely reviving a method invented by Hippocrates. But this claim was inaccurate. Hippocrates had developed a method of shaking the patient in order to hear the fluid moving inside him. Yet others ridiculed Auenbrugger's innovation. They called it a molestation of the sick. Only one favorable review appeared in a medical journal. The reviewer called Auenbrugger's discovery "a torch that was designed to illumine the darkness in which diseases of the thorax had up to this time lain concealed."[2] Overall, Auenbrugger's work attracted little of the attention it deserved.

This did not discourage Auenbrugger, however. Futile resentments or the pursuit of an acrid controversy had no place in his life. He simply continued his medical practice with the conviction of a man certain of the truth and utility of his work. Over the years, he was much in demand as a consultant for ailments of the chest although other doctors did not often practice his methods. Auenbrugger understood that new ideas are accepted only with time and with difficulty. He continued a successful professional and private life. He was well-liked in the cultural circles of Vienna. He was a personable man, whose avocation and music delighted many. He once wrote a light opera, The Chimney Sweep, which became very popular. When the Empress asked him his reason for not writing another he answered that one was enough. When he was sixty-two, he was knighted by Empress Maria Theresa because of his personal popularity.

Forty-seven years after the publication of *Inventum Novum,* the personal physician to Napoleon, Jean Nicholas Corvisart, translated Auenbrugger's booklet. The Austrian doctor's technique rapidly came to world-wide attention thereafter, and even today remains a basic diagnostic method.

BACON

"More secrets of knowledge have been discovered by plain and neglected men than by men of popular fame. And this is so with good reason. For the men of popular fame are busy on popular matters."[3]

                                                  Roger Bacon

A medieval English philosopher and scientist, Roger Bacon (c. 1220-1292), was early interested in the classics and the disciplines that comprised the quadrivium—geometry, arithmetic, astronomy, and music. He received two Master of Arts degrees, one from Oxford and another from Paris. While in Paris he was preoccupied with philosophy, particularly Aristotelian teachings, and with theology, both of which became his chief concerns.

But in 1247, Bacon's intellectual interests and habits changed considerably because of the influence of several English scientists. Instead of involvement with the commonly accepted scholarly interests, he now pursued natural science and experimental research. He was fired by the desire to find truth. He was tired of the unthinking repetition of principles expounded eleven centuries before him. This blind acceptance of dogma inherited from the ancient Greeks rankled him. He acquired special equipment and books that cost him a considerable amount of money, and he worked long hours with his research. He began a series of experiments in diverse fields of knowledge. From this research he wrote treatises on optics, which suggested the construction of spectacles for those with poor sight, predicted modern inventions, such as horseless carriages and flying machines, demonstrated that light travels faster than sound, experimented with chemical analysis, computed the inaccuracy of the Julian calendar, and performed countless other investigations.

In 1257, Bacon entered the Franciscan Order of Friars Minor in a quest for peace. But the Franciscans soon found the maxim by which Roger lived blasphemous: "Look at things, try them, see how they can act on you, and *how you can act on them.*"[4] Searching into God's secrets was not man's business. And trying to change nature was even worse. Bacon was constantly under suspicion for heresy. He did not help his lot by his openly voiced contempt for those who did not share his zeal.

In 1266, Bacon wrote several letters to Pope Clement IV, a former acquaintance, referring to some of his progressive knowledge in education, church affairs, and science, and his projected reforms in these areas. Thinking that Bacon had actually written an encyclopedia of knowledge, the Pope ordered him to send the manuscript to him for further study and to avoid telling others of the work. Undaunted by this request for something that did not yet exist, Bacon set to work and in very little time wrote the *Opus majus,* the *Opus minus,* and the *Opus tertium.* He did so secretly. But his irregular conduct made him suspect to his superiors who watched him yet more closely. The *Opus majus* was a persuasive document, written in hopes of convincing the Pope to institute various educational and church reforms. Bacon sent this manuscript to Europe with one of his favorite pupils. But travel was very slow, and the manuscript did not arrive until after the Pope's death. It then fell into complete oblivion for the next four and a half centuries, not to be published until 1733.

Although discouraged by this mishap, Bacon did not relinquish his research which, because of his medieval credulity, led him to investigate and sometimes embrace superstitious arts, such as astrology and alchemy—both considered by the church to be magical arts denounced by God. His fellow Franciscans suspected all of his teachings and grew bitter at his condemnatory attacks on leading theologians and scholars. Sometime between 1277 and 1279, he was condemned to prison for heresy. There he remained until 1290 when a new Pope was elected. Of his difficult life he wrote this:

I believe that humanity shall accept as an axiom

for its conduct the principle for which I have laid down my life—the right to investigate. It is the credo of free men—this opportunity to try, this privilege to err, this courage to experiment anew. We scientists of the human spirit shall experiment, experiment, ever experiment.[5]

Not long after his release, he died, but his death went unnoticed and the death date is thus uncertain.

As has been true for many great men, Bacon's contributions were discovered after his death. Suddenly he was named "doctor admirabilis." Exaggerated accounts of his accomplishments were written for the public. Fantastic stories of building and rarifying bridges in the air and of strange experiments with magical mirrors became part of his popular image. Proper appraisal finally came, however, when he was accepted as a great philosopher who had advanced science through his ceaseless crusade for the experimental method. Bacon himself assessed the importance of work when he stated that "experimental science has three great advantages over all other sciences; it discovers truths which would never otherwise be found; it examines the course of nature, and it makes possible knowledge of the past and the future."[6]

BLACKWELL

> "... all the gentlemen I meet seem separated by an invisible, invincible barrier and the women who take up the subject partially are inferior. It will not always be so; when the novelty of the innovation is past, men and women will be valuable friends in medicine, but for a time that cannot be."[7]
>
> Elizabeth Blackwell

Elizabeth Blackwell (1821-1910) was born in Bristol, England. From early childhood she encountered unconventional ideas. Her father was a church dissenter, and because of this, she was not allowed to attend the respected schools supported by the Church of England. So she and her brothers and sisters received their education from tutors. In 1832 the Blackwell family moved to America, eventually settling in Cincinnati, Ohio. They became acquainted with the more forward-thinking people of their age—people involved with abolition and the women's rights movement. When Mr. Blackwell died, the oldest children started earning money to support their family of ten. Because little else was available to educated women, the oldest daughters opened a boarding school for young women. Later when their brothers were well enough established in business, they closed the school. But Elizabeth, very concerned with the problems of education for women, continued her involvement in teaching and tutoring. One day, a friend dying of cancer suggested that she study medicine. At first, Elizabeth did not even consider it, but she could not seem to escape the idea. She finally decided to attend medical school; a woman had never done so before. She taught for several years to earn tuition fees while studying privately with sympathetic doctors who lent her medical books and guided her studies. She applied to major medical schools. But her applications, if answered, were always rejected. Often they were just ignored. Friends encouraged her either to disguise herself as a man in order to enter the formal study of medicine or to travel to Europe where schools reportedly accepted women. But Blackwell refused to give up her moral crusade. "A course of justice and common sense," she wrote, " must be pursued in the light of day."[8]

Instead she obtained a list of smaller schools and sent applications to twelve of these. All answers were negative, as she had almost come to expect, except for one small school, Geneva University. In the acceptance letter the dean of the faculty welcomed her, stating that certainly she could "elevate (herself) without detracting in the least from the dignity of the profession." He wished her success in her endeavor, "which some may deem bold in the present state of society."[9]

Interestingly enough, the faculty actually had not wanted her to attend their school but had been too embarrassed to reject her application which had been accompanied by a letter from an eminent Philadelphia physician. Instead they decided to let the students bear the responsibility of rejection. They referred her application to the student body stipulating, to ensure rejection, that just one negative vote would veto Blackwell's attendance. But the class, well-known for its unruliness did not agree with the faculty. After laughter, cat-calls, handkerchief waving and hat throwing, all chorused "Aye" at the voting, with the exception of one faint "Nay." "On the instant the class arose as one and rushed to the corner from which the voice proceeded. Amid screams of 'cuff him' and 'crack his skull,' a young man was dragged to the platform screaming, 'Aye, aye, I vote aye.' A unanimous vote in favor of the woman student had been obtained by the class."[10] A formally stated resolution was quickly sent to the faculty, notifying them of the decision, although imparting no suggestion of how it was reached.

Blackwell was well-accepted at this university. The formerly riotous class was transformed "from a band of lawless desperadoes to gentlemen."[11] The faculty soon accepted her too, although she did meet up with a few perplexing situations. An anatomist, Dr. Webster, requested that she not attend his lectures on the reproductive system. She replied, politely but firmly, that "the study of anatomy was a serious one ... All branches of it reflected glory on the Creator. She could not therefore imagine that a dedicated man of science would be disturbed by the fact that student No. 130 wore a bonnet. But if it would distract him less, she would be delighted to remove her conspicuous headgear and sit in the back row."[12] Dr. Webster became her loyal supporter. The university administration also temporarily stood in her way. They were afraid to be the first school to confer a doctor's degree on a women. But when they learned that Blackwell had earned the highest average on the examinations, they awarded her the degree of Doctor of Medicine.

The Geneva townspeople did not accept Blackwell so readily. They ostracized her, considering her either mad or disreputable. But their reaction to her was just a foreshadowing of her future treatment. Blackwell went on to complete her training at Blockley Hospital. There, the other doctors openly avoided her. They did not write down the patients' diagnoses or treatments, purposefully complicating her work.

Seeing that a medical degree was not enough to help a woman set up a practice, Blackwell traveled to England and France to continue her studies. She was well received in London, but in Paris she was barred from studying in the hospitals. She was only allowed to enter an obstetrical center that trained mid-wives. There she was treated like the eighteen-year-old girls who came for training. The senior intern, Hippolyte Blot, however, befriended her, showing her special cases, instructing her, and introducing her to exciting medical advances. Later that year, she suffered a great setback that forced her to give up surgery. She was treating a baby with ophthalmia and accidentally infected her own left eye. For three weeks she lay in darkness with both eyes closed. The sight in her left eye was permanently lost, but after special treatment and a rest in the mountains of Germany she was able to retain the sight in her right eye.

She returned to England. In London, she was given permission to study in any ward of St. Bartholomew's Hospital but the department of female diseases. She attended lectures and met many leading medical men. She also met Florence Nightingale, at this time a young woman with dreams but no means to fulfill them. The two often discussed their futures as women in medicine.

Blackwell returned to the United States in 1851. She decided to establish a practice in New York City. But landladies refused to rent a room for that purpose. Finally she rented the entire floor of a boarding house because she was told that no one would share a floor with a female doctor. After she notified the neighborhood of her practice, she began to receive abusive letters. Her practice had no chance. So she tried to join a hospital staff, but none would accept a woman.

Finally she started a lecture series on the physical education of girls which she advertised in the *New York Times*. A small audience of intelligent and influential men and women welcomed her advanced ideas. Soon Blackwell had a very small practice of wealthy women. But she was dissatisfied because she wished to help the poor. With some financial help she opened a small office in one of the most indigent areas of the city where she treated the sick three days a week. These times were very difficult and lonely for Blackwell: "I had no medical companionship, the profession stood aloof, and society was distrustful of the innovation. Insolent letters occasionally came by post and my pecuniary position was a source of constant anxiety."[13]

In 1856, her sister Emily finished her medical studies in Edinburgh under Sir James Simpson, Queen Victoria's obstetrician. Emily traveled to New York City to work with her sister. Another young women, Marie Zakrzewska (called Dr. Zak), whom Blackwell had assisted, also finished her education in 1856. Now Blackwell had two doctors to help her. After much planning and fund-raising the women opened the

New York Infirmary for Women and Children in 1857. They rented and fixed up a house on Bleecker Street in Greenwich Village. It was opened in May by the Rev. Henry Ward Beecher and various prominent physicians who approved of the women's work.

This hospital was the first completely run by women. Because of this it had troubles. It was stormed two times by angry crowds who would not accept it. Then it had tremendous financial difficulties. For many years, its income depended on the three women's extra efforts: bazaars, lectures, concerts, and any other means of fund-raising were pursued. The doctors continued their work, serving three thousand patients the first year and many more after that. Sometimes they had help from other women doctors newly graduated who needed the opportunity to gain practical experience at the infirmary.

In 1858 Elizabeth Blackwell returned to England after transferring directorship of the dispensary to her sister. She had always longed to practice medicine there. The Medical Act of 1858 allowed physicians with foreign degrees to register without examination if they were already practicing medicine in England. Blackwell registered shortly before the deadline. She was the first woman doctor recognized in England.

She returned to America to help found a medical school for women. The school reflected some important advances in medicine and medical training: hygiene was a major subject, previously little considered; an examining committee independent of the faculty was formed; the term of study was lengthened from three to four years. After the school was launched, Blackwell returned to England. Her sister directed both the infirmary and the medical school from 1869 to 1899. Elizabeth Blackwell, until her death in 1910 at the age of eighty-nine, devoted her life to writing and lecturing about medicine.

Blackwell did not live to see the day when men and women could become valuable friends in medicine, but she deserves full credit for having opened the doors of the medical profession to women.

BOYLSTON

"Obstinacy and vehemency in opinion are the surest proofs of stupidity."[14]

Bruce Barton

The first American medical publication that we know of is "A Brief Rule to Guide the Common People of New England on How to Order Themselves and Theirs in the Smallpocks, or Measels" by Thomas Thacer. Its appearance is readily understood when we learn that smallpox, the colonists' most feared scourge, had come from Europe with them and between the years 1683 and 1702, had broken out eight times. In Boston in 1721 smallpox appeared once again. Cotton Mather, the prominent and distinguished Puritan minister, remembered reading an article in the Philosophical Transactions of the Royal Society about two doctors, Timoni and Pylarini, in Constantinople, Turkey, who had successfully inoculated people against smallpox. He also remembered a slave who had told him about African tribal practices similar to inoculation. Although Mather, a stern Calvinist, had always believed that disease and pestilence were God's just chastisement of man, he now saw his own children in danger and willingly accepted the hope of possible prevention. He approached some of the Boston physicians with his findings. But they just denounced the crazy notion of inoculation, saying that "the Novelty of seeking Security from a Distemper, by rushing into the Embraces of it, could naturally have very little tendency to procure it a good Reception on its first Appearance."[15]

But Dr. Zabdiel Boylston listened to Mather's proposal. Boylston (1680-1766), the eldest son of a doctor educated in England, acquired his education from his father and Dr. John Cutter, an eminent Boston physician. Boylston soon became a respected doctor noted for his kindness toward and concern for his patients. He also gained some distinction as a naturalist through his correspondence with Sir Hans Sloane, president of the Royal Society and a well-known naturalist. His curiosity in the sciences led him to consider and adopt Mather's idea. He decided to lay his plan for inoculation before other physicians, hoping to gain their support. But he didn't anticipate William Douglass's violent opposition. Douglass, an obstinate and arrogant man, had been educated in Edinburgh and Paris. In fact, he was the only colonial doctor who had actually earned the degree of Doctor of Medicine. Colonial America had no formal training for doctors. Because of his position he never acknowledged personal errors and he disliked those whose discoveries might outstrip him. He called on a friend, Dalhonde, a French physician, to denounce Boylston and Mather and their proposal for inoculation saying it would only spread the plague. The two began a series of publications against inoculation. Later Dalhonde even filed a legal deposition against inoculation. In it he told gruesome tales of men in Italy, Flanders, and Spain, who had died horrifying deaths from gangrened colons, tumefied organs, livid diaphragms, ulcerated lungs—all because of inoculation. Then some of the more conservative clergymen began to preach against inoculation. Men are defying God's will, they said as they condemned Mather for abandoning Calvin's principles.

Soon Boston's citizens became enraged at Boylston and began to patrol the town, threatening to hang him. At one time the threats grew so numerous that Boylston had to go into hiding in his own home for two weeks. Parties of men came and went, searching his house, but never finding him. His family was also abused. One night while his wife and children were sitting in the parlor, someone tossed a lighted bomb into the room. Fortunately the fuse was knocked off; otherwise the family would have been killed.

Despite this violence, Boylston decided to commence inoculation. He started with his own son, thirteen years old, and two slaves, one thirty-six, the other just two years of age.

After a week he knew that his experiment had succeeded; the three patients had survived. Having soothed some of the fears, he secretly began to inoculate 247 patients. Two other doctors who supported Boylston inoculated thirty-nine more. Of these 286, only six died (2%). Three of these were said to have contracted the disease before inoculation. During this same time, 5759 contracted smallpox without inoculation; 344 of these died (14.6%). And many who survived were disfigured and chronically ill.

Boylston's announcement of his success only rekindled the people's anger. He was summoned before the town council, as he would be many times in the next year, to answer for his actions. Repeatedly he asked physicians to visit his patients and to judge the worth of his unorthodox work. But they refused. Instead, they passed resolutions saying that inoculating smallpox "has proved the death of many persons for the natural tendency of infusing such malignant filth in the Mass of Blood."[16] They then introduced a bill into the legislature that prohibited inoculation. Luckily it did not pass because of some of the councilmen's doubts.

The controversy continued and publications began to play a major role. James and Benjamin Franklin, printing and editing the *New England Courant,* denounced inoculation and clergy who encouraged it. Soon these clergymen became the target for popular abuse. Some were insulted and physically injured on the streets, and even their worship services were disrupted. Mather himself was attacked. A bomb whose fuse also fell off was once thrown through his window with a note attached reading, "Cotton Mather, I was one of your Meeting; But the Cursed Lye you told of—You know who; made me leave You, You Dog, and Damn You, I will Enoculate You with this, with a Pox to you."[17]

Then Dalhonde's deposition was printed and the people became so furious that Boylston was prohibited from continuing his work although he did so secretly and even in disguise. Boylston then published a defense of inoculation in pamphlets and in the *Boston Gazette*. Some clergymen who agreed with him published tracts and books defending inoculation. Others, particularly John Williams who advocated the death penalty for those who inoculated, answered these defenses with their own pamphlets which tried to convince Bostonians that inoculation was the devil's invention to rid the world of Christians. One said:

> I do not see how we can be excused from great impiety herein, when ministers and people . . . make supplications to Almighty God to avert the judgement of the smallpox, and at the same time some have been carrying about instruments of inoculation, and bottles of the poisonous humor, to infect all who were willing to submit to it, whereby we might as naturally expect the infection to spread, as a man to break his bones by casting himself headlong from the highest pinnacle.[18]

The published defenses and attacks and the threats of violence continued unabated until the disease lessened and disappeared.

After the epidemic ceased and the controversy died down, Boylston received an invitation to England from Sir Hans Sloane. The two men had been corresponding during Boylston's difficulties, and Sloane, very curious about inoculation, wished to hear more. In England Boylston was cordially and respectfully treated despite the occasional misrepresentation of his work which followed him even to England. He was elected into the Royal Society—the first American to receive this honor—and he was introduced to the royal family. During the next year and a half, he met many other distinguished scientists and doctors. Before his return to America in 1726, the Royal Society asked him to publish a tract on his method of inoculation.

In the Colonies Boylston resumed his medical and scientific pursuits. Men like Douglass still harassed him, but to little end. After many years Boylston retired from his profession and pursued agriculture. He died in 1766 at the age of eighty-six.

The controversy over inoculation continued with each outbreak of smallpox for the next thirty years. But slowly people began to accept the preventive approach to it. Even Benjamin Franklin, who had so bitterly opposed it, later said that he regretted not having allowed his son to be inoculated. His son died of smallpox when he was only four years old.

D'ABANO

"In this matter, however, some mischief makers, unwilling or rather unable to hear, for a long time have freely vexed me, from whose hands at last the said truth has laudably snatched me and mine, with the intervention, too, of an apostolic mandate."[19]

Pietro d'Abano

Pietro d'Abano (1250-c. 1315)—the first professor to give Padua its distinguished reputation, an excellent physician, and a famous philosopher—can be regarded as one of the last medieval men of science. Coming at the height of this revival, and also its close, Pietro saw his work as compiling, supplementing, and correcting his predecessors' work. He studied, and translated into Latin, the works of great physicians and scientists. Important writings of Aristotle, Galen, Mesue the Younger, and many others could finally be read in Latin. Pietro's greatest work—*Conciliator differentiarum philosophorium et praecipue medicorum* (1303)—dealt with medical issues, dispelling contradictions so much a part of medical tradition. The first part concerned general questions; the second, theory of medicine; and the third, its practice. A problem would be presented, followed by quoted theories and opinions of the great authorities. Then the argumentative section balanced the pros and cons to discover the truth and resolve the contradiction. The correct doctrine remained in the end.

The questions discussed varied greatly: Does air have mass? Does blood alone nourish? Is there a mean between health and illness? Is pain felt? Does the pulse contain musical consonance? How often should a person eat? Should one exercise before or after meals? Does confidence of the patient in the physician assist recovery? Is paralysis of the right side harder to cure than paralysis of the left side? Does milk agree with consumptives? Some of these questions are still being asked. Pietro's *Conciliator* attempted to reconcile the differing opinions on many issues of physicians and philosophers who had lived before him.

In order to research these men and their opinions, as well as other topics, Pietro traveled widely—to Sardinia, where he studied a poisoning; to Constantinople, where he discovered a volume of Aristotle's Problems that had never before been translated; to Venice, where he visited with Marco Polo; perhaps even to Spain, England, and Scotland although there is no proof of this. Much of his life, however, he spent at the University of Paris where he was called the "great Lombard." While there he discovered the writings of Abraham ben Ezra, a well-known astrologer who lived in Spain in the 1100's. The existing translation of his writings from Hebrew was poor, so Pietro published a more reliable rendition of his own. In studying these writings, Pietro became very interested in both astronomy and astrology. He included in his books discussions of history—the rise of religions and prophets, etc.—with its relationship to the course of the stars and the planets. These bold inclusions aroused considerable opposition and gave competitors, envious of his remarkable success as a physician, a reason to oppose him. Many accounts even tell of a trial by the Inquisition in 1306 in which Pietro was charged with heresy in practicing magic and disputing Christianity. According to Savonarola, Pietro was saved by the King and by the university who so venerated him. Historians are not sure whether Pietro faced the Inquisition again, but they are sure he was persecuted because of various allusions to these difficulties in his writings. Presumably Pope Boniface VIII issued an injunction in Pietro's behalf.

Shortly thereafter, Pietro returned to Padua to hold a prominent position at the university. He continued his writing, his practice, and his teaching, helping the school gain its reputation as a leading medical school. Little is known of Pietro's activities in the years to follow, but certainly he continued his interest in astrology and philosophy, for the Church watched him carefully. Thomas of Strasbourg, who was prior general of the Augustinians from 1345 to 1357, called Pietro a heretic, although a most capable physician, who disbelieved the New Testament miracles, claiming that the dead who were raised had only been in a trance.

Pietro realized that his skeptical thinking was dangerous and tried to protect himself. In his last will and testament he professed a firm faith in Christianity and the Church, adding that "if it should be found that he has ever said anything contrary to the Faith, he said it not because he believed it, but probably for purposes of disputation."[20]

This profession, however, did not protect him. Again, some sources claim he was tried before the Inquisition for heresy in 1315. But he died before the trial's conclusion. Pietro was pronounced guilty. His body was exhumed and burned. Thomas of Strasbourg stated, "I was present when in the city of Padua his bones were burned for these and his other errors."[21] Later sources claimed that friends hid Pietro's body so that the Church burned an effigy in the public square. Another source tells of a faithful maid who hid his body and then had it buried in the church of St. Peter at Padua. Savonarola does not mention the Inquisition, but rather a Dominican inquisitor so enraged that "in the dead of the night opened the sepulchre, burned the body, and gave the ashes to the wind. O unspeakable crime!"[22] Although no one knows the exact circumstances surrounding Pietro's death and later exhumation, it is certain that he was persecuted in his later years, and that either his corpse or an effigy of him was burned.

After his death his reputation as a magician and a heretic became less important as scholars could reflect upon his many accomplishments. Of the 182 medical books printed before 1481, eight were Pietro's. Pietro D'Abano was also an outstanding teacher, scholar, and practitioner who helped to reconcile many different viewpoints. More than a century after his death, Frederick, Duke of Urbino, recognizing Pietro's contributions, had the doctor's effigies set up over the gates of the palace of Padua with the inscription: "Peter of Abano and Padua, most learned in philosophy and medicines, and on that account winner of the name of Conciliator; in astrology indeed so skillful that he incurred suspicion of magic, and, falsely accused of heresy, was acquitted."[23] Thus Pietro d'Abano was accorded the praise he was due more than a hundred years too late for him to appreciate it.

GALEN

"The price we pay for our great men is that later generations make tyrants of them."[24]
                                Sir Thomas Clifford Allbutt

Claudius Galenus, known to us as Galen, was a Greek born in Pergamum in 130 A.D. His father, afraid that his son would inherit his mother's argumentative nature, named him "Peaceful One" or "Galen" in an attempt to influence his character. But Galen never was the peaceful one. His life was full of conflicts and dangers; and even after his death his ideas were the source of conflict for centuries.

Galen's father was persuaded by a dream to direct his son into medicine. So after several years of philosophical studies, Galen began four years studying anatomy at Pergamum. He then traveled to Smyrna and Corinth where he worked with the most eminent men of his day. Early he developed an infallible memory and accurate powers of observation. He soon flaunted his knowledge with great self-assurance. He felt himself qualified to judge any aspect of medical science.

At the age of twenty-nine, he returned to Pergamum where his practice started out with flourishing success. He was clever in surgery and careful in his prescriptions, so that patients traveled from neighboring villages and islands just for his help. During the summer sports season he was appointed physician for the gladiators. He set sprains and fractures and dressed wounds, always washing them with red wine first. The first year no one died of injuries—a great achievement. He retained this position for four years. But when the Galatians attacked Pergamum, the games ended, and Galen saw in this an opportunity to improve his status. On the edge of the empire he could at best become a local celebrity. For fame and wealth he would need to go to the capital.

Galen moved to Rome in 163 A.D. at the age of thirty-three. But life in Rome was vastly different from life in Pergamum. Life was rough and undisciplined. He found his colleagues to be malicious and ignorant. But he was given his first chance to prove his skills when he was asked to treat a philosopher suffering from a fever. Galen treated him and then predicted when the fever would lift; miraculously his prediction came true. Suddenly the superstitious Romans began to hear of a physician who had magical powers. His name was mentioned in the highest circles. At first the wealthy, as a precaution, just sent their slaves to be treated. But soon patricians flocked to him for advice.

During this first flurry of success, his supporters persuaded him to hold public lectures. At these lectures Galen demonstrated vivisection of pigs and then proceeded to discuss his many theories, at the same time discounting the Sophists, the Methodists—any scientific or philosophical group he disagreed with. Some of his listeners were impressed by his self-assured manner and confident speech, while others took offense.

Court physicians and their Roman colleagues could not endure the sight of this Greek physician receiving all the honors and later the fees which once flowed to them. They began to heckle and slander him and even considered resorting to physical harm. At one point Galen was afraid of being poisoned. He was forced to give up his public lectures and instead began a prolific writing career. He began to amass the medical knowledge physicians until his time had gathered. He also began many experiments and dissections. Over the years he dissected many animals—pigs, goats, dogs, bears, fish, birds, and monkeys. The last he considered the most valuable because of their resemblance to humans. He dissected only two human bodies, both badly decomposed by the time he received them.

But through his experiments he began to answer questions men had often asked. He attempted to explain the circulation of blood. Erasistratus had taught that air flowed through the arteries. But Galen proved that blood, not air, flowed through the arteries. The blood, he said, was pushed into the arteries by the left ventricle. But then he had to explain what happened to the pneuma—the air-like substance—that was supposed to be circulating through the body too. The pneuma was believed to pour from the lungs into the left auricle and ventricle? But then how did the blood get into the left ventricle. Galen theorized that it came from the right ventricle through the muscular partition between the two by way of tiny holes. He went on to conclude that the difference between the color of blood in the left ventricle and arteries, and right ventricle and veins was due to the presence of pneuma from the lungs. He incorrectly concluded that the blood streamed in all directions, although the valves prevented flow reversal.

With his experiments and successful practice, Galen came to the attention of the Emperors, Verus and Marcus Aurelius. He was given permission to hold a lecture on his new discoveries. But at this time rumors spread of a ghastly epidemic brought back by soldiers returning from the Parthian Wars. Galen realized that this epidemic could in short time destroy his reputation, if not kill him. And so he left suddenly for his home city, cancelling his lecture. The epidemic broke out with unbridled force in Italy.

Marcus Aurelius and Verus returned to Italy to inspect their troops and in desperation sent for Galen who, after several delays and a lengthy journey, finally could find no excuse to prevent his return to Italy. At the imperial headquarters at Aquileia the plague was at its worst. Emperor Verus died while fleeing this camp. In an attempt to avoid remaining there, Galen persuaded Marcus Aurelius to allow him to travel back to Rome with the remaining Emperor's ill son Commodus. Galen was able to diagnose the child's illness correctly and cure him. Because of this he was appointed physician at court. He spent what little free time he had on the voluminous writings he stored in the Temple of Peace which later burned, resulting in the destruction of many of his manuscripts. But he had no time for experimentations as patients came to him from the farthest reaches because of his great reputation. This reputation Galen owed not only to his comprehensive knowledge and experience but also to his ability to inspire faith in his treatments. Galen was the fashionable physician whom scores of people sought for advice and cures.

But when Commodus became Emperor, he put a stop to visits from Galen, saying he had no use for his magic. This left Galen to his many projects. After Commodus' assassination, Galen was once more the fashion. Only this time he waited on the new Emperor's wife who had him concoct all sorts of beauty preparations.

After these many years of practice, there was no aspect of the body Galen had not spoken on and in so doing he had prescribed many health practices. He had advocated exercise, gymnastics, and hunting, cold baths for the young, and warm baths and wine for the old, pork for athletes, and dyes, paints, and perfumes for women. In his five hundred treatises of various lengths, he had covered many subjects from ethics, logic, and grammar to anatomy and surgery. He had answered all questions without hesitation or doubt. He was the Great Galen who had triumphantly marched against ignorance and stupidity. When he died in 201 A.D., no one dared question his statement that "Anyone who, like me, aspires to become famous for his deeds rather than for pompous speeches, must relentlessly absorb everything which I have stated after a lifetime of hardworking research."[25]

Certainly Galen thought very highly of himself. But how was it that he gained universal acceptance as the dictator of medical knowledge for fourteen centuries? Even into the seventeenth century his works were quoted and defended, usually without further research. The reason for his power lay perhaps in the fact that his writings, particularly his fourteen-volume book *On the Method of Healing,* supplied physicians with a compendium of medical art and science with commentaries and additions written with such convincing assurance that physicians believed his claim that he had finished what Hippocrates had begun. This consolidation of medical knowledge was valuable, but all too soon it became an obstacle to progress because Galen's word held undisputed sway.

His studies of human anatomy which were based on animal dissections and supposition became the texts for medical schools. Sometimes his statements were correct; other times they were false. For example, he recognized that inspiration was associated with enlargement of the chest. But then he went on to state that air passed inside the skull carrying off humors from the brain. He could not let loose of the various traditional doctrines: the humoural beliefs of Hippocrates which classified diseases as due to yellow bile, black bile, phlegm, or blood; and the doctrine of the four elements—fire, air, water, and earth with their combinations of heat, cold, dryness, or moistness. He was also greatly involved in dispensing medicines, including amulets, which he classified according to their elemental qualities not their therapeutic effects. For all of his practices he constructed an elaborate logical system of medicine that combined many of his beliefs: the complexions, the temperaments, the four elements, the four humours, the Critical Days (a remnant of magical numbers), etc.

Many of these beliefs kept medicine in fetters for centuries. On the other hand, Galen made many valuable contributions. He investigated the effects of environment on health and disease. Like many physicians today he believed that for someone to become ill the victim had to be in a receptive condition. Through his skillful dissections, he discovered the function of motor nerves; he learned that blood flows through the veins and arteries. He taught the value of topographical anatomy. The list of his successes is lengthy. But most of all, he was the greatest master of scientific method, some say, until Roger Bacon. If physicians had adopted his methods of inquiry and research, they would have been able to arrive at the truth. Instead they latched onto his words and without further investigation held them in such great reverence that only a few brave doctors ever experimented and researched to discover their validity. Those who actually proclaimed a different truth from Galen's were for centuries ignored, mistreated, ridiculed, and sometimes even hunted down and killed. True, Galen was a remarkable and intelligent scientist; but those who blindly followed his ideas succumbed to the tyranny of believing that he and they knew all the answers.

GOLDBERGER

"They are thrown into a state of mental fog and confusion if you cannot instantly explain every reported epidemiological observation...They reason that inasmuch as I cannot explain every observation that therefore, I must be wrong."[26]

Joseph Goldberger

In the early 1900's, an explosive outbreak of pellagra in the southern United States forced the Public Health Service to direct more support and attention to this problem, the cause of which had already been debated for more than a century. With forty-one men assigned to study pellagra from various approaches and $80,000 allocated to the first year of research, Joseph Goldberger accepted the appointment to head the project.

Goldberger (1874-1929)—a Jewish immigrant born in Hungary—grew up in New York City. He first decided to study civil engineering. But, after attending a medical lecture by chance, he dropped engineering and entered Bellevue Hospital College from which he graduated with honors in 1895. After two years of practice, he was bored. He joined the Public Health Service, which sent him first to Ellis Island, then to Mexico, Cuba, and later Puerto Rico. At all of these locations he studied infectious diseases, such as yellow fever and typhus fever. The expertise he developed earned him the assignment to work on pellagra in the South.

Goldberger surveyed the studies under way and toured the South to see the extent of the problem. In particular, he observed mental asylums and other institutions. After less than five months on this project, he announced that the problem was dietary and urged people to eat more fresh meat, milk, and eggs. To substantiate his statement he conducted an experiment with two orphanages in Jackson, Mississippi. Sixty percent of the children at one of these had pellagra in early 1914. Goldberger recommended more fresh protein which the government helped to buy. A year later the health of the children was better than it had ever been. But the superintendent of one orphanage in sending out his annual plea for food for the children's home asked for molasses, flour, sugar, corn, grits, cured meats, and canned goods. Even after having seen the benefits of a good diet he was willing to return to the former diet. Goldberger moved on to other orphanages to test his diet treatment. The results were successful. Some orphanages learned from the experiment; others didn't. A healthy diet seemed possible when supported by the government. But without this aid, administrators returned to the old, less expensive dietary patterns.

Meanwhile, Goldberger was facing opposition from fellow health officers and physicians. At the Southern Medical Association's meeting in 1914 and at one of the meetings of the Association for the Study of Pellagra in 1915, he got a taste of things to come. His ideas were either laughed at or not acted upon. This reception grew much worse when he announced the results of a secret research project in which he produced pellagra in healthy white males by feeding them a poor diet. The Governor of Mississippi authorized the experiment for Rankin Prison Farm and promised to pardon any dozen men who participated. The convicts at the prison were in good health. In fact, Rankin Prison Farm had never had a case of pellagra. The twelve volunteers were fed a diet of mostly refined and simple carbohydrates: polished rice, corn meal, flour, sugar, molasses, sweet potatoes, collards, turnip greens, pork fat, and coffee. Quite early the men started to show symptoms of pellagra, however the disease could not be diagnosed as such without the tell-tale dermatitis. After five months skin lesions finally appeared and four experienced physicians confirmed the diagnosis of pellagra in six of the men. Twenty years later scientists learned that dermatitis resulting from pellagra depends on the action of sunlight on the skin. The prison volunteers had been kept indoors, thus explaining the lengthy time before the skin lesions developed.

News of the experiment hit both the local and national press. Some praised Goldberger's breakthrough. But many objected to his work. Medical men were angry because the research had been done in secret. Others were angry because of the implication of Goldberger's theory—that the South was starving its people. Everyone could see the strong association between poverty and pellagra. One doctor even observed that the best prevention of pellagra was $200 in the bank. But at numerous meetings, one speaker after another rejected Goldberger's diet theory for the old favorites. They blamed pellagra on all sorts of causes: corn bread, amoebas, sugar, infection, the stable fly, Italian immigrants, etc. James A. Hayne, South Carolina's Health Officer, became Goldberger's most vocal opponent and a good representative of what Goldberger called the "impressionistic school" of research in which the researcher, in his comfortable chair, gazes out the window for a time and then announced his impression of scientific data.

Criticism of Goldberger's work appeared also in books published after the prison experiment. Some criticized Goldberger's research technique, others, his diet theory. One doctor emphasized his belief that pellagra was caused by soft or freestone water common to clay soil districts. He even sent a letter to Governor Brewer deprecating Goldberger's ideas and praising his own. The Governor responded that the doctor should produce pellagra by using freestone water and he would be convinced.

Overall, the men who attacked Goldberger resented him as an outsider who was finding too much fault with the South and who was disagreeing with everything they had been taught about the germ theory. Goldberger's work was ahead of its time. Doctors did not know that deficiencies in certain chemical substances could cause disease. It was not until after 1915 that physicians even began to look at nutrition. To them, this was the chemist's domain.

Goldberger decided to spike the arguments of his germ-theory opponents. He designed an unpleasant experiment in which he attempted to transmit disease from a pellagrin to a healthy person. Goldberger, his wife, and fourteen associates took part in this project. Seven times they tried to contract pellagra using every method they knew of infection: blood, nasal secretion, urine, feces, scales from skin lesions, etc. At the "filth parties" several got mildly ill but no one contracted pellagra. When Goldberger announced his experiment, the infectionists quieted down a little but still objected to his theories. The Pellagra Commission of the National Medical Association even stated that pellagra is a communicable disease, suggesting poor sanitation as the culprit. Other researchers and physicians also suggested causes: larva in the soil, alcohol, heredity, etc.

Although many attacked Goldberger's theory, others ignored him. A comprehensive work on pellagra by Henry F. Harris did not even mention Goldberger's name. Although, the doctor was beginning to gain the support of the nutrition authorities, these men did not have the support of traditional medicine.

In 1916 he launched an important study of several communities to prove pellagra's relationship to diet, diet's determination by the Southern economy, and the Southern economy's dependency on a one-crop system. The failure of a cotton crop could upset any Southern community's perilous economy. And this took a toll on the community's health. Reports of Goldberger's findings in national newspapers published in 1920 again wounded Southern pride. Their poverty and increasing problem with pellagra was being paraded before the nation. But their anger did not peak until President Harding saw the article and took action. In a letter given top billing in newspapers, the President discussed the problems of famine and disease, promising legislative action if they were not controlled. The South vigorously protested: "Famine does *not exist* anywhere in the South...and we fail to find evidence of a general increase in pellagra."[27]

Southern political leaders as well as Southern health officers denied that pellagra was increasing. Businessmen feared that the President's letter and the attention given to the South would ruin their business interest. Articles from different sections of the South extolled the region's bounty. Very few Southerners urged their fellows to welcome aid and education for the people.

When Goldberger called a meeting of the state health officers, agricultural experts, and relief agencies to devise a plan of action, he was hit by the furor of the Southern health officers who charged him with slander so that even the President would state that the South was haunted by famine and disease. These outbursts continued at other meetings.

Goldberger, outwardly calm, was inwardly outraged at their stupidity—"blind, selfish, jealous, prejudiced asses,"[28] he called them. To put their negativity to rest he knew he needed to isolate the nutritive ingredient that prevented pellagra. He returned to the laboratory with a new associate, W. F. Tanner. First, they worked with amino acids, finding tryptophan important in treating pellagra. But within several months they began to search for a vitamin. Time was to reveal a special relationship between tryptophan and the pellagra-preventing vitamin. But they had yet to discover the vitamin. These next years were years of quiet research, minor criticism, and some praise.

The previous years of virulent opposition had told on Goldberger. Paul de Kruif, bacteriologist and author called him a "soft-spoken desperado." Goldberger realized his work had not even dented the problem because of poverty and human ignorance. "After all, I'm only a bum doctor, and what can I do about the economic conditions of the South?"[29] he said.

In 1927 medical organizations began to accept Goldberger's diet theory, even pledging support to agricultural agencies. But the doctor remained skeptical; social and economic changes were needed before pellagra would ever be eradicated. Eventually his recommendations were put into practice and the rate of pellagra declined for the first time in years. Goldberger did not live to see this. Nor did he live to find the vitamin he searched for. He died of cancer in 1929. After his death his work was attacked because his work was incomplete. Through the work of many researchers, nicotinic acid, described as a chemical in 1867 and isolated by Fank in 1912 from rice polishings, was identified as the anti-pellagra vitamin.

Yet pellagra continued to haunt the South because so many refused to believe it existed. How could the South, how could America, have a hunger problem? "I doubt if they are any worse off in Belgium,"[30] Goldberger wrote of the people of South Carolina mill villages during World War I. "Some day this will be realized and something done to correct it."[31]

GRODDECK

"I am a wild analyst."[32]

Georg Groddeck

Georg Groddeck (1866-1934), born in Baden-Baden, Germany, studied at Kaiser Wilhelm University in Berlin. One of the professors there, Ernst Schweninger, an eccentric and tyrannical doctor, became Groddeck's mentor. Schweninger, who was greatly involved in physiotherapy, taught Groddeck to doubt claims he could not personally prove, to disparage any drug or device that did no demonstrable good, and to regard the physician as a mere catalyst, initiating healing only. These unorthodox teachings became the basis for Groddeck's future work.

After eight years of service in the army and marriage to a young divorcee with two children, Groddeck began work in Schweninger's sanitarium with such success that he was able to open his own sanitarium with his sister's help. He spent the rest of his life at this clinic. Much of his early practice dealt with diet and physical therapy, including massage. But he was not satisfied with this.

Because of a disappointing marriage and a restless search for a more meaningful pursuit, he began a writing career. Over the next forty years he wrote novels, essays, literary criticism, and a defense of Schweninger's methods that attacked the new psychoanalysis of Freud. But then he made an exciting discovery that changed his life.

He undertook the treatment of a woman who suffered from several diseases and who had tried many different treatments. She was close to death, and because of this, Groddeck listened attentively and kindly to her. He soon was aware that she was unable to say stool or stovepipe, and she could not tolerate objects, such as the chamber pot and the footstool, in her room. She was also greatly embarrassed when people absently pulled at their nose or ear lobe or twirled a pencil.

After a week of discovering which movements, objects, and words were forbidden, he began to understand her mental world. Because of his involvement in literature, he was aware of symbols. But this was his first experience with a patient who confused symbol with reality. He soon realized the women's inability to deal with bodily functions. The stovepipe represented the male; the stovebox, the female. And absentminded gestures represented masturbation. The stool took on another meaning as well. By the time the woman left the sanitarium, she was in far better health than she ever thought possible because she understood some of her problem.

Groddeck tried this same listening and watching game with other patients and began to see the power of symbols in many of his patients. He began also to ask questions: What was the power of emotions? How did the attitude of the patient to the physician affect recovery? What were the meanings behind random or habitual gestures? Were patients unknowingly willing to be ill? Why were eighty percent of his patients women?

And so Groddeck moved slowly into a new field of medicine. His medical practice had always been successful but now his growing reputation as a wonder doctor began to attract patients from all over Europe. He did not understand his success with the new psychotherapy until he changed his definition of illness. No longer was illness just a physical dysfunction of the body, but rather a symbol created by the patient.

After another brief stint in the army which resulted in dismissal from his post because he had angrily protested interference in his methods, Groddeck returned to his sanitarium where he continued his practice, coming closer and closer to many of Freud's theories through his own observations. In 1917, he wrote to Sigmund Freud, describing some of his cases, and then presenting his idea of *Das Es,* the It:

> Long before I met the above-mentioned patient in 1909, I was firmly convinced that the distinction between mind and body is only a word, not an essential distinction—that the body and mind are a joint thing which harbors an It, a power by which we are lived, while we think we live...I have tried to treat the whole individual, the It in him: I have searched for a way leading into my untrodden, the pathless. I knew that I was moving closer to the borders of mysticism, if not already standing in the very thick of it.[33]

Freud was impressed by Groddeck's attempt to restore the concept of unity in many and to treat the body through the mind. Groddeck was not just propounding a theory; he was practicing it, and with success. Freud wrote to Groddeck: "Everything that comes from you...is interesting to me, even if in the details I am not always in agreement. In your *It* I do not recognize my civilized, bourgeois *Id*...However, you know that mine is derived from yours."[34] And thus began the correspondence and friendship between the two men until Freud's death.

This friendship with Freud was particularly important to Groddeck, not because physicians now felt they could accept his radical ideas—they ignored and laughed at him—but rather because he could now publish his views. He soon published the first investigation into what today is called psychosomatic illness. Many of his ideas in this pamphlet were controversial and surprising to his fellow-physicians. But Groddeck was always careful to call for further testing of his claims. He too was uncertain about the field he was entering. He also introduced his concept of the It:

> Just as the It affects the senses, it also affects the digestive processes, the distribution of blood, the activity of the heart—all in all, the total organic life of the personality is being constantly changed. In the same manner this It protects itself against

> the threat of all chemical, mechanical, and bacterial attacks, and by the same token it may, when illness seems advisable, produce conditions in which the pathological germ can be permitted to be effective.[35]

Groddeck's theory of the It was the major theme in all his articles, and he did not change the concept in his remaining years.

At this time Groddeck also decided to apply for membership to the Berlin Psychoanalytic Society. Overall he was not welcome because of his odd theories and practices. But, according to rumor, Freud influenced the group to accept Groddeck. And at the International Conference at the Hague, Freud persuaded the Society to allow Groddeck to deliver some words on the subject of his pamphlet.

Groddeck mounted the platform, and the first words he uttered were "I am a wild analyst." If these words did not alienate the group, the speech that followed did. He did not read a prepared paper; he simply gave a demonstration of free association, rambling from one topic to another. He enjoyed stirring people up, especially these psychoanalysts who considered him a crank.

Shortly after this experience, he worked on two important books. One was the first psychoanalytical novel, *The Soul Searcher*. But he could find no one who would publish it because it was quite shocking. Because Freud admired it, it was later published by the Psychoanalytic Society. Another important work was *The Book of the It*. In this he wrote freely about his analysis of himself, discussing his envy of woman's ability to bear children, which he believed caused his problems with goiter. Only when he learned of his unconscious pregnancy fantasy did his goiter disappear.

> Our unconscious expresses itself in symbols: in love for God, crime, and heroism, good deeds and evil ones, religion and blasphemy; in staining the tablecloth and breaking glass; in the invention of

tools and machines; in art, sickness, and death—in every aspect of our lives...The doctor has two questions to decide: By what means is the It contriving to remain sick, and by what means can it again be induced to want to be healthy?[36]

Groddeck also published a paper on the relationship between dreams and organic symptoms. And in his last work, *Man as Symbol,* he discussed art, language, sickness, and their use as symbols for man. He claimed, for instance, that the true artist is not a spectator or a master; he is an interpreter of the It—the unconscious. And this It exists long before the brain develops, revealing itself ever afterwards in one's bodily functions, in his profession, age, schooling, marriage, etc. Man, however, masters the It, arranging and organizing, and completing, forming the *I* which stands over against the It.

These ideas were heatedly debated. Groddeck was either praised or condemned. No middle ground existed. Not until he turned sixty did Groddeck receive any official tribute for his work, and this he received only because a good friend wrote it. Those who applauded him were the rebels who did not care about others' opinions. And Groddeck was right in the thick of these rebels.

During his last years, Groddeck refused to believe Hitler was anti-semitic. He believed Hitler's colleagues were responsible for the outrages. He wrote Hitler several times in an attempt to influence his actions. But this only endangered his own life. Frieda Fromm-Reichmann arranged a lecture for Groddeck in Switzerland and he traveled there to speak despite serious heart trouble. He collapsed after the presentation and died several days later.

The controversy over Groddeck's theories which began in his lifetime continues today. Some of his pupils practicing psychotherapy even asked that their names be in no way associated with their teacher's. Groddeck's ideas were often too daring, too speculative. Some physicians who accepted his ideas never practiced them. Many doctors now accept the idea that emotional stresses can cause physical symptoms. But they do not use the logical reverse that Groddeck preached and practiced: That emotions can heal the body. Doctors talk about lowered resistance without delving any further to understand some people's propensity to illness.

But these controversies about Groddeck's thought are infrequent today because so few have ever even heard his name. An examination of major works on psychosomatic medicine, of which Groddeck was the founder, turned up very few works that even mention him. And those that do, give him but slight reference. And so Groddeck's contributions to psychoanalysis and psychosomatic medicine have yet to be recognized. His theories deserve careful consideration and testing. Some, like his theory of childbirth without pain and his recognition of emotional factors in hypertension, heart disease, ulcers, etc., have already made reputations for other physicians. Perhaps one day Groddeck's thought will be well researched so that he will be given proper c edit for many innovations and for his place as the founder of psychosomatic medicine, a term he disliked because it still perpetuated the dichotomy between body and mind.

HARVEY

"These views as usual pleased some more, others less; some chid and calumniated me, and laid it to me as a crime that I have dared to depart from the precepts...of all anatomists."[37]

William Harvey

Physicians in the Middle Ages had no clear conception of the blood's movement in the body. They did not conceive of it as circulating continuously in one direction, returning to its point of origin, the heart. Instead, they thought that blood, starting in the liver, moved slowly and irregularly in any direction and at any speed. They did not view the heart as a muscle, but rather as an organ that expanded because of pulsating animal spirits. They believed it had pores in its septum that allowed blood to seep from one ventricle to the other.

Early in his career, William Harvey (1578-1657) began his study of the vascular system. He discovered that the valves in veins allow blood to flow only toward the heart while the arteries allow blood to flow only away from the heart, circulating it through the entire body. He also showed that the heart (whose septum has no pores, he found) is a pump, and that, through expansions and contractions, moves the blood through the body. Harvey demonstrated his findings when he lectured in London in 1616, and in subsequent lectures, always adding further evidence and proof. He was able to find time to continue his experiments and lectures after he was appointed court physician to James I in 1618 and later to Charles I. When he was fifty, he decided to publish his long-tested conclusions in the quarto, *Exercitatio anatomica de Motu Cordis et Sanguinis in Animalibus (1628)*.

His ideas were so revolutionary that he and his teachings were fiercely attacked by numerous physicians. Primrose, a Galenist, said that Harvey could not find the septum pores because the septum changes upon death. Others, like Hofman, would not accept the heart as a muscle. Guy Patin of Paris called Harvey's theory "paradoxical, useless, false, impossible, absurd, and harmful."[38] Harvey's most violent adversary, Jean Riolan, claimed that Galen could never be wrong, although perhaps man's body had changed since Galen.

Other physicians simply ignored Harvey's work. Thomas Winston, who certainly knew of Harvey's ideas and had heard him lecture, never mentioned Harvey's teachings in his writings. A colleague of Harvey's, Alexander Reid, in his *Manual of Anatomy* completely ignored the new ideas. Jean Riolan the Younger and Descartes tried to reconcile Harvey's and Galen's theories, resulting in ridiculous conclusions that in- cluded such assumptions as the heart's pumping only one or two drops of blood each hour. Then there were those who tried to deprecate Harvey's discoveries by pointing to previous physicians, like Servetus and Caesalpinus, who had made initial discoveries in circulation. Harvey's own statement that no man over forty years of age accepted his theories is pro- bably a fairly accurate judgment of what happened.

Soon many others entered the argument: naturalists, philosophers, and even clergymen, who were reluctant to view the heart, much spoken of in the Bible, as a mere muscle. With such a negative reaction, it is not surprising that Harvey's practice suffered. A friend of his, John Aubrey, wrote, "I have heard him say that after his booke of the Circulation of the Blood came out, that he fell mightily in his practize, and that twas beleeved by the vulgar that he was crack-brained; and all the physitians were against his position and envyed him."[39]

Even eight years later when he traveled to the continent, Harvey met with indignant protest from various physicians who observed his demonstrations and experiments and yet refused to believe his conclusions. No evidence exists showing that on this trip Harvey visited Padua, where he had studied medicine. If he did visit, he arrived incognito so that he would not have to face the certain censure of those still teaching and studying Galen. Like many others, they regarded Harvey as a traitor.

Harvey was able to endure his losses because of wealthy relatives and because of his position as court physician. His theories were also supported and proven by various respected doctors and scientists. Despite this support, his theory was often attacked over the next twenty years. Harvey only once published a defense in answer to these attacks, finding his time more profitably spent continuing his teaching and studies. Twenty years later he issued a second edition of his work.

Harvey's problems were soon magnified by his royalist sympathies. No longer were the English satisfied with Catholic Charles I. In 1642, Cromwell and his Puritan supporters, the Roundheads, were beginning their campaigns against the Royalists. Popular opinion turned against all Royalists. Once, while Harvey was away from London to meet with a colleague, his home was ransacked. His collections of butterflies, chrysalises, worms, embryos, skeletons—a scientific collection that had taken him years to assemble—were broken and his manuscripts scattered and destroyed. Harvey fled with Charles I to Oxford, returning to London after the King's execution in 1649. But he no longer had the strength to continue his work as before. His wife was dead, his king had been executed, his practice was gone, and his home was destroyed. Henceforth, he lived with one or another of his brothers. During these years he helped the Royal College of Surgeons in establishing a library and a museum. And he was persuaded to publish a last book on embryology, *De Generatione Animalium* (1654) which he did not wish to publish because of the possibility of raising controversy once again. But a friend, after much argument, was able to convince him of the work's importance.

Harvey lived to see his discoveries accepted in many universities. His observations, which were explanations of the body's functioning, opened the door for further research that would lead and is still leading to amazing development in understanding human functioning.

HICKMAN

"People who will attack any innovation, however true and beneficial it may be, always have existed and always will exist."[40]
                                    Sir William Hale-White

    Sir Astley Paston Cooper related an experience that occurred before the discovery of anesthesia. His uncle, surgeon William Cooper, was preparing to amputate a man's leg. The patient arrived in the operating theater. But after one look at the instruments he lost all courage and rushed out of the hospital. "William Cooper made no attempt to recover him; he merely remarked, 'By God! I am glad he is gone!' "[41]

    This reaction to the escaping patient was perhaps more common than we would expect. To operate on a patient while he suffered great pain must have been trying. Nonetheless, the discovery of anesthesia was a slow process due partly to the church's belief that suffering was part of God's will for fallen mankind and therefore should not be relieved. The French in the seventeenth century even passed a law forbidding the use of drugs to relieve pain.

    Not until the start of the nineteenth century did surgeons begin to consider inhalation anesthesia. Humphrey Davy in 1799 breathed in nitrous oxide and suggested its use during surgery. But his proposal received little attention. For years this gas and sulphuric ether were used for their exhilarating qualities. Young people carried bladders of "laughing gas" or bottles of ether to parties sometimes called "ether frolics."

    Then in 1820 an Englishman, Henry Hill Hickman (1800-1830), began what soon became a large country practice. Often he amputated limbs, removed kidney stones, repaired hernias, and performed tracheotomies. He worked quickly but could not avoid causing pain. The notion that pain was inevitable, which he had always rejected, led him to the theories of Beddoes, the founder of pneumatology, which had been discredited if not forgotten. He experimented with a puppy which he placed under a glass dome. The puppy after approximately fifteen minutes was unconscious, and Hickman was able to cut off one of its ears without inflicting pain. Hickman realized that the animal's state was due to suffocation but he thought that some other gas—perhaps laughing gas—could be used without harming the subject. So he continued his experimentation with success.

Soon he wrote of his findings and theories for their application to humans to a scientist who passed them on to Sir Davy. Davy was too busy with his own work and no longer cared to hear about laughing gas and its possible uses. Hickman then published a pamphlet presenting his experiments and proposing that a similar procedure could render human beings insensible to pain. No one seriously considered his ideas. In fact, after reading a paper on his experiments before the Medical Society of London, he was laughed at and called "a dreamer, not to say a fool" and a "danger to the faculty."[42]

Hickman then wrote to Charles X of France asking to demonstrate his procedure. His letter was referred to the Royal Academy of Medicine which called a meeting for its review. Only Baron Larrey, surgeon of Napoleon's armies, considered Hickman's discovery, offering himself as the subject for the demonstration. But the Academy, ridiculing Hickman's "crazy scheme" outvoted Larrey, declining to have anything else to do with this innovation.

Hickman finally returned home discouraged but unwilling to give up his struggle for the alleviation of pain. But he died prematurely several months later at the age of 29. His work to ease unnecessary pain had been slighted by those who feared innovation.

HIPPOCRATES

"...the disciples of Hippocrates had elevated the teachings of their master almost into a religion, and were bound far too closely to his authority, to the exclusion of original thought and progress."[43]

Sir James Elliott

Very little is known about Hippocrates, the father of medicine, and what little is known is surrounded by legend. Various accounts of his life exist but the one most trusted is thought to be a chapter from Soranus' *Lives of Physicians*. Hippocrates was born about 460 B.C. during the golden age of Greece at Cos. He was trained in medicine by his father and later by Herodicus. Other accounts claim he was also trained by Gorgial the rhetorician and Democritus the philosopher, evidence for which can be found in the Hippocratic Corpus. There was a very famous medical school at Cos which owned an extensive library considered the authoritative collection of medical knowledge. Hippocrates studied there as well as in other Greek towns, particularly Athens. He quickly became known for his keen observations. Because of these he was the first to state that disease is the result of a natural and intelligible cause. He recognized Nature as the healer, the physician as her servant, and the patient as an active participant in the healing process. Before too long he was reputed to be the greatest physician in Greece.

When his parents died, Hippocrates left Cos. Some sources suggest he left because he set fire to the Cos medical school library, although he supposedly said that he wished to visit other places and further educate himself. Perhaps the rumor of his setting fire to the library was the result of envious colleagues in Athens who accused him of vanity and selfishness. Many Athenian physicians were from the Cnidian School of medical thought which opposed the Hippocratic School in quite a few of their theories.

The stories of his travels certainly exceed probability, although they are not impossible for a well-known physician. It is written that Hippocrates was invited by the King of Macedonia, who was suspected to be suffering from consumption, to reside there as a court physician. While there Hippocrates discovered that King Perdiccas was in love with his dead father's concubine. Hippocrates told her of Perdiccas' love and in the end he was cured. Hippocrates was then summoned to Abdera to cure Democritus of insanity and to save the city from an epidemic.

Another source records that the great physician was invited to two countries north of Greece where the plague had broken out. But when he discovered the prevailing winds were from the north, he refused their offer because he was certain the plague would reach Athens and other city-states. This was typical of meteorological medical beliefs many held. But Thucydides states that the plague came from the south, so this story is probably further from the truth than others.

Hippocrates is said also to have been wooed with promises of great wealth to attend the court of the Persian Artaxerxes. But Hippocrates, out of patriotism, declined the generous offer. One source, the pseudo-Hippocratic Letters, includes a decree from the Athenians praising Hippocrates for sending his pupils throughout Greece during the times of plague, for successfully treating it, for publishing medical books for all physicians, and for remaining true to Greece in refusing the Persian offer. In return he was to be initiated at no personal cost into the Eleusinian mysteries, to be crowned with a golden wreath, to be given Athenian citizenship, and to be allowed sustenance for life. None of these details can be confirmed, but they suggest the great respect and veneration, accorded the Greek physician.

Hippocrates died at Larissa in Thessaly at a great age recorded as anywhere from eighty-five to a hundred and nine years. He left two sons, Thessalus and Draco, well-known in their own rights, and many pupils. He also left a great collection of writings. The authorship of these has been constantly debated. No uniform style exists in these writings and no authors' names are given for the treatises. No firm conclusions have even been made about works that are the genuine writings of Hippocrates. One authority's conclusion seems the most likely: the books are part of a library belonging to the master physician of a medical school. The collection was given Hippocrates' name because he was its collector and first owner. Scholars do not know which books, if any, were written by Hippocrates. Therefore to try to divine his style and personality in the books is useless, although they clearly contain his doctrines.

Much of Hippocrates' medical practice was based on his theories of the humours, of temperaments, and of pneuma. The four humours—the fluid constituents of man—were blood, phlegm, yellow bile, and black bile, each different in color, dryness, and warmth. Each prevailed in the different seasons of the year and were also affected by diet. For example, Hippocrates stated that phlegm, characteristically white, increased in winter as it was the coldest fluid. It could be seen in sputum, nasal discharges, etc. When a humour was excessive, treatment had to be set against it. If a patient had too much blood, the excess was drained away with leeches.

The theory of the four humours was directly linked to that of the temperaments. Although the humours changed seasonally, man was ruled by one of the humours temperamentally. The familiar classification of phlegmatic, sanguine, choleric, and melancholic dispositions was created. The temperaments affected constitution and health in different ways.

While the humours represented the fluids in man and determined his physical makeup, his health and his disposition, the pneuma represented the gases or air in man and accounted for his consciousness. These theories of pneuma and the humours were the foundation of Greek medicine, as anatomy is the foundation of modern medicine. Dissection of human bodies was forbidden on religious grounds, so that the

Greeks had no conception of circulation or the nervous system. The Hippocratic Corpus does contain some anatomical passages particularly about bones; most of this knowledge probably came from observation of both the injured and uninjured and from inspection of skeletons. In fact, Hippocratic surgery dealt almost solely with bones and their accompanying tissues.

Although the Hippocratics understood little about the body and the causes of disease, they were able to develop clinical treatment. Hippocrates' ability to observe began a new era in medicine. He said that "the best physician is the one who is able to establish a prognosis, penetrating and exposing first of all, at the bedside, the present, the past, and the future of his patients, and adding what they omit in their statements."[44] This called for excellent observation at which Hippocratics excelled with close attention to the patient's appearance, behaviour, breathing, sweating, temperature, and excretion.

The diagnosis was made on the grounds of physical appearance and past experience recorded in close studies of the visible process of disease. Before treatment was decided upon, the physician was to decide whether he should treat the patient or not. The Hippocratics were cautious and gentle in all they undertook, and they refused to accept desperate cases. This would make them laughingstocks, and physicians held too unstable a position to allow the stigma of failure.

Treatment included matters such as rest, comfort, washing, warming, and diet, and on the psychological side, sympathy and encouragement. These therapies were discussed in a series of books on regimen. This consisted primarily of diet and exercise. These had to be decided upon with attention to the season, the winds, the individual's age, and his home situation. Regimen in disease added the various interventions allowed: first, medicine; second, the knife; and third, the fire. What the fire could not cure was considered incurable.

From his experience with observation and treatment of disease, Hippocrates went on to classify diseases as sporadic, epidemic, and endemic. He also separated acute from chronic disease. And he divided disease into general causes—climate, water, sanitation, etc.—and personal causes—diet, exercise, etc.

But Hippocrates was not solely interested in treatment of disease. Among the Greeks the concept of positive health was current. They did not consider it preventive medicine, which was a negative view of health. They wished to maintain positive health, not to avoid illness, to have the highest quality of health possible, which they often viewed as an aesthetic characteristic. Excellent health was the physical counterpart of mental cultivation sought after by man, not just by athletic competitors or warriors. And so Hippocrates spoke to the development of positive health with various regimens also.

In his regimens and therapies, Hippocrates was not afraid to discuss his failures and his doubts. He was courageous in that he defied medical tradition when he saw no reason for it, and that he was not afraid to openly discuss ideas. After his death, however, his disciples so elevated his teachings that they bound medical progress. His teachings were quoted by Plato, Aristotle, Galen, and various Arabic writers. Hippocrates' spirit of openmindedness was not emulated. He would have welcomed progress, and yet, ironically, his teachings barred the door to progress for centuries.

LAVOISIER

"La Republique n'a pas besoin de savants; il faut que la justice suive sa course."[45]

            Coffinhal

Antoine Lavoisier (1743-1794), sometimes called the father of modern chemistry, studied law as a young man but left these studies when he became more interested in science. With another scientist he prepared a mineralogical atlas of France that won him an election into the Royal Academy of Sciences. He then began a series of reports on various topics, such as an analysis of gypsum, explanations of the aurora borealis and thunder, and a refutation of the belief that water could be distilled into earth. He also wrote technical reports for various industries: mines, soap factories, iron works, etc. He even won a gold medal for a paper on a lighting system for a city.

He then, rather surprisingly, accepted a position in the Ferme Generale, a private company that aided the government in tax collection. He worked there for the next twenty-three years, eventually securing a top administrative position. Nonetheless, he was able to spend several hours each day on his own scientific studies. His young wife, who was devoted to him and his work, illustrated his articles, translated English scientific articles into French for him, and helped with his experiments. During this time Lavoisier also served on various committees. He wrote reports for the committee on agriculture, instructing farmers in agricultural betterment. He also helped to standardize weights and measures and to develop the metric system. He submitted ideas to the government for improvements in many areas, such as hygiene, public education, coinage, cannon casting, taxation, and pensions. But his service as director of gunpowder was perhaps most helpful to him because he was given a house and laboratory in the Royal Arsenal where he could continue his experiments.

Lavoisier's most important discovery concerned combustion and oxidation. Scientists believed that when something burned, it lost phlogiston so that the substance remaining was the same as the original except that it no longer contained phlogiston. This loss explained the weight difference between a lump of coal and its remaining ashes. But Lavoisier could not accept this theory because he knew that some calcined substances gained weight. Priestley, an Englishman who discovered oxygen without realizing it, once visited Lavoisier and described the newly discovered gas's properties. Lavoisier knew that this gas was the key to his problem. He experimented with sulphur and phosphorus, finding that they gained weight when calcined because they absorbed this "vital air." Other substances lost weight upon calcination because they lost the "air." Lavoisier eventually called this new gas "oxygen" (meaning "acid-maker") because he mistakenly assumed that it could be found in all acids. But he did discover that combustion was not the liberation of phlogiston but the combination of oxygen with a burning substance.

Lavoisier then went on to explain respiration. He and Pierre Laplace experimented with an ice calorimeter, measuring the heat produced by respiration. They found it was similar to the heat produced by slow combustion when the same amount of oxygen burned charcoal. Respiration resulted in the blood's absorption of oxygen used to burn food for the body's energy, and expiration of carbon dioxide. Lavoisier thus solved the long-standing puzzle of breathing—a puzzle that had always intrigued William Harvey. He then applied his discoveries to practical needs, insisting on adequate air space for people forced to live in close quarters, and calling for the abolishment of dungeons.

Lavoisier with his followers then developed a new system of naming substances by their constituents. The existing nomenclature was not based on any rational system. The compound "vitriol of Venus" was called "copper sulfate" with Lavoisier's new system. Developments like this allowed chemistry to become a true science.

During these last years of Lavoisier's experimentation, the French Revolution started. Those who were associated with the previous government were under immediate suspicion. In 1791 the Ferme Generale was closed. This affected Lavoisier but not as much as another difficulty. He had once stated that a scientific article on combustion written by Marat was meritless. This had greatly angered Marat who now saw his opportunity to strike back at Lavoisier. In his newspaper, *L'Ami du Peuple,* he condemned Lavoisier as "King of charlatans, companion of tyrants, pupil of scoundrels, master of thieves."[46] He also accused him of plotting for election as administrator of Paris. He then called for Lavoisier to be hanged from the nearest lamp-post. Lavoisier ignored the article. But Marat continued his attacks against the scientist.

In 1793, all learned societies were suppressed, including the Academy of Sciences which Lavoisier now directed. When he objected to this suppression, he was charged with treason. Then he and twenty-seven former employees of the Ferme Generale were arrested and sent to the prison of the condemned. The trial was brief. All were charged with plundering the French citizens and the national treasury, supplying France's enemies with this money. Lavoisier was also charged with watering the tobacco supply and with stopping the circulation of the air in Paris by advising the erection of a wall around the city. When someone spoke up in Lavoisier's defense, mentioning his many contributions to science and to France, the judge, Coffinhal, stated that the "Republic does not need the learned; she must follow the course of justice." For all his supposed crimes, Lavoisier was called a vampire to the people of France and then sent to the guillotine. One observer, Lagrange, whispered to a friend, "Only a moment to cut off his head, and perhaps a century before we shall have another like it."[47]

After Lavoisier's death and the deaths of many other scientists, those responsible for the supplies needed in the revolutionary wars realized that they had guillotined the ones whom they now needed. France lacked gunpowder, cannons, saltpeter, steel, and many other provisions. The Republic could no longer claim she had no need for the learned.

LISTER

"A man laid on the operating table in one of our surgical hospitals is exposed to more chances of death than the English soldier on the field of Waterloo."[48]

                Sir James Young Simpson

Someone once described the surgeon in the early 1800's as a medieval peasant who sowed his seed and then waited resignedly to see what God would allow the harvest to bring. All too often the harvest was death. As the number of surgeries increased, so did the number of deaths. The mortality from septicemia, gangrene, and erysipelas was appalling. This fact distressed Joseph Lister (1827-1912), who early in his medical career at the Royal Infirmary of Edinburgh was astonished at the paucity of knowledge about inflammation. He was convinced that something in the air brought about suppuration, although he did not agree with many doctors that the gases in the air were the cause. These same men would demolish and rebuild whole hospitals in order to be rid of "bad air."

Lister started his research by describing the first stages of suppuration: heat, redness, swelling, and pain. He and other scientists still hoped to control disease through learning about its natural history. Neither the germ theory of disease nor the idea of infection had been introduced. And observations were as yet superficial and confused. During Lister's early career, Ignatz Semmelweis's futile attempts to combat childbed fever had already been forgotten. In fact, Lister did not even hear of the Hungarian's work for another twenty years. Lister was working in a time when little was understood about the body and the advances made were often rejected.

Fortunately Lister heard of a French chemist who was conducting interesting experiments with wine and beer fermentation. In the 1860's he read of Louis Pasteur who was proving that fermentation was not the result of chemical action as most believed, but rather the result of tiny living germs—micro-organisms. When Lister read this news, he saw its medical implications. An outside cause—germs in the environment—was responsible for suppuration.

He then set to work to test this theory. He knew that somehow he needed to kill the germs. Pasteur recommended heat, filtration, or antiseptics. Lister chose an antiseptic, carbolic acid. Although his first antiseptic solutions and dressings were quite crude, in time he improved his technique. By 1867 he published an account of his work with compound fractures and the use of carbolic acid in *The Lancet*. In this article he explained a complicated technique that needed to be followed. This system was under continuous development for the next twenty years, and it involved many details: the strength of the acid solution, its mode of application; the types of dressings, their size, the frequency of their changing; precautions in dressing wounds; preparations for surgery, etc. All of these depended on particular circumstances. Physicians reading all these directions were boggled by the seeming complexity of Lister's method because they didn't understand its consistency with the underlying germ theory.

Gradually physicians here and there began to try his system. The results were mixed. Some thought his precautions ridiculous and simplified his method, thus deleting its effectiveness. Once the editor of *The Lancet* wrote that "Mr. Lister's treatment does not find much favour in London. Are the conditions of suppuration different here from those in Glasgow or Dowlais? Or is it that the antiseptic treatment is not tried with that care without which Mr. Lister has always pointed out it does not succeed?"[49] Other doctors found the system quite successful. Numerous letters began to appear in *The Lancet,* speaking for both sides of the issue.

As the advocate for this new surgical principle, Lister had several disadvantages. First, he was not a personable man; he was rather aloof, a trait some historians claim was due to a stuttering problem he had as a boy. Although he was always kind and considerate, he was also very grave and quite unapproachable. Second, Lister was not a controvertialist. He believed all too readily that reason would eventually prevail and so did not often argue his point. Because of this, many doctors unfamiliar with his system assumed that all it consisted of was splashing the wound with a little carbolic acid. They would then write to *The Lancet* with news of the failure of antisepsis.

One of Lister's major opponents made this assumption and, because a French surgeon had once recommended the use of carbolic acid, claimed that Lister was simply appropriating another's ideas. This attack came from Sir James Young Simpson, who apparently had forgotten the battles he himself had fought in defense of chloroform anaesthesia.

In 1869, Lister's father-in-law, James Syme, resigned the Chair of Clinical Surgery in Edinburgh and Lister was elected to the vacant position. This period was probably the brightest of his career. He was able to revolutionize the surgical wards of the Royal Infirmary and in so doing his fame was well-established in Scotland and abroad. In Denmark, Sweden, and Germany, his ideas were researched and found valuable. But in England, especially London, his assertions were questioned, mocked, and ignored. During this period, Lister successfully toured Europe with his ideas, but this did not help to persuade the London doctors to assess his work with more openmindedness. Again they attacked him; this time asking for statistical evidence of the efficacy of his system. One doctor cited sixty-three amputations resulting in only three deaths and twenty-three joint excisions resulting in two deaths for the old system, and then he demanded Lister's results. However, Lister was performing surgeries never before attempted because it was assumed the patients would die of suppuration. His supporters chided him for not reporting many of these surgical advances, but he refused because he knew that other surgeons would attempt the same operations and would lose their patients to sepsis. Beyond that, Lister's statistics could not be compared to amputations and joint excisions.

Finally Lister saw his chance to personally introduce his antiseptic system to London when he was invited to fill the Chair of Clinical Surgery at King's College in London. He accepted the post but was not prepared for his reception. Lister took with him four assistants because no one at the hospital had been trained in antiseptic techniques. The five doctors felt as though they were campaigning in enemy territory. The hospital wards were almost empty and the staff was at best indifferent to the changes being forced upon them. But the greatest problem came with the nurses, the Sisters of St. John. The nurses' despotism at King's Hospital was complete. They were the authorities on cleanliness and on the rules of conduct. They hampered Lister and his assistants as much as they could. They required special forms before anyone could be admitted for care or could be carried to the operating theater. These requirements resulted in near-death situations for some of Lister's patients who needed emergency help.

Lister was also poorly received in the classroom. One day while he was lecturing on the fermentation of milk, attempting to show evidence for the new germ theory, the students shuffled their feet, mooed every time he said the word "cow," and when the bell rang they shouted, "Tea-time." This distressed Lister but not nearly as much as the poor showing at his lectures. Once no one showed up. The students had quickly discovered that the material Lister taught was considered balderdash and when they used it on their examinations they were failed.

Lister's major problem at the college lay in convincing his older fellow-physicians to accept his ideas. They refused, perhaps because his system would antiquate their skills. With antiseptics, more complex surgery was possible. They would go from experienced surgeons to beginners in little time. And they would be replaced by the scientifically trained youth moving into their ranks.

But as Lister continued his teaching and his practice, people began to see the effects of his system and his practices were gradually accepted. He had more battles to face with regards to the germ theory, but by 1880 most of the opposition had disappeared. However it was not until 1897 the *The Lancet* finally declared that "Listerism is destined to be the surgery of the future."[50]

By this time Lister had already received countless honors—honorary degrees from Oxford and Cambridge and numerous foreign universities. By 1912, the year of his death, he had been awarded a baronetcy and a peerage, an honor no other medical man had yet received. He was also president of the Royal Society and in a meeting with Pasteur at which he was presented the official greetings of the Royal Society, he spoke of the debt surgery owed to Pasteur. Perhaps he regarded this moment as the most memorable in his life. Because of Lister's insight and dedication, surgery entered a new era.

MCDOWELL

"A great theory has never been accepted without opposition. Such must always be the course of things so long as men are endowed with different degrees of insight; where the mind of genius discerns the distant truth which it pursued, the mind not so gifted often sees nothing but the extravagance which it avoids."[51]

Professor Tyndale

Surgery in America first became a specialized area under the influence of Philip Syng Physick. The University of Pennsylvania abolished the chair of anatomy, midwifery, and surgery and established a separate position for surgery. Physick first held this professorship because of his fine reputation as both a surgeon and a teacher. He also invented and improved several surgical instruments. But surgery as of yet included no gynecological surgery and little abdominal surgery. The pioneer in these fields was Ephraim McDowell (1771-1830).

McDowell received his medical education from practical experience with Dr. Alexander Humphreys and from the University of Edinburgh, where he worked especially with Dr. John Bell, an outstanding professor. When McDowell returned to Danville, Kentucky, in 1795, he quickly established himself as the best surgeon west of Philadelphia.

But his first opportunity to gain fame did not come until fourteen years later in 1809. Two physicians asked his advice about a patient, Mrs. Jane Todd Crawford, who was late in delivering twins. McDowell examined her and discovered a large tumor. He explained the situation to her, saying that the tumor needed to be removed, but its removal meant almost certain death. Mrs. Crawford decided to risk the surgery, traveling sixty miles on horseback in the winter, resting the tumor on the saddle's pommel.

With the assistance of his nephew who had studied some

medicine and his apprentice, McDowell began the operation. Outside a crowd of angry, excited men who had heard that McDowell was going to "butcher a woman" awaited the results of the operation. If the patient died, the doctor would be responsible and would pay with his life according to harsh frontier justice. Inside Mrs. Crawford lay on a table reciting psalms while McDowell opened her abdomen, ligated the tube, and removed the tumerous ovary which weighed almost twenty pounds. The intestines had fallen out after the incision was made and became so cold during the half-hour surgery that McDowell bathed them in tepid water before replacing them. He then sutured the incision and put the patient to bed.

Only five days later, Mrs. Crawford was making her own bed, and twenty-five days later, she traveled home to live thirty-one more years. McDowell considered publishing news of his amazing surgery but realized physicians would not believe that he, a frontier doctor, could successfully perform an operation which they would not even attempt. Besides, he wasn't sure whether to attribute the success to luck or skill. So, he decided to wait until he had more experience with the surgery.

In 1813 and 1816 he again successfully performed the operation. He then sent an account of the three cases to Dr. Physick. But this celebrated surgeon could not conceive of a backwoods doctor accomplishing the impossible. He would not have it published. So McDowell sent the article to Dr. Thomas C. James, head of the midwifery department at the University of Pennsylvania. James, most interested in the account, published the article in 1817 in his journal, *The Eclectic Repertory*. The response was disheartening. The general reaction was disbelief and dismissal. Two surgeons who wanted to attempt McDowell's procedure wrote letters blaming the deaths of their patients, on whom they were afraid to operate because of the inadequacy of his description of the procedure.

McDowell answered these charges in a letter to Dr. James,

stating that his description had been clear and detailed enough for any able surgeon. And he hoped no other would attempt the operation:

> It is my most ardent wish that this operation may remain, to the mechanical surgeon, forever incomprehensible. Such have been the *bane* of the science; intruding themselves into the ranks of the profession, with no other qualification but boldness in undertaking, ignorance of their responsibility, and indifference to the lives of their patients; proceeding according to the special dictates of some author, as mechanical as themselves, they cut and tear with fearless indifference, utterly incapable of exercising any judgement of their own in cases of emergency; and sometimes, without even possessing the slightest knowledge of the parts concerned. The preposterous and impious attempts of such pretenders, can seldom fail to prove destructive to the patient, and disgraceful to the science. It is by such this noble science has been degraded in the minds of many to the rank of an art.[52]

McDowell then added news of two more ovariectomies. One patient had recovered; the other had died of peritonitis. McDowell also sent a letter explaining his new surgery to Dr. Bell at Edinburgh University, but it was not published until 1824 in the *Edinburgh Medical and Surgical Journal*. By the end of his career, McDowell had performed twelve or thirteen ovariectomies with only one fatality—an excellent record for his time.

He originated other minor operations, but he did not report them. McDowell is also credited with performing successfully the first cesarean section in America; he did not report this either. But he did travel to Europe three times to do cesarean sections. And his reputation as a surgeon was so great that he was asked to operate on President Polk to remove bladder stones and repair a hernia.

Although McDowell was much praised in certain circles for his contribution to surgery, he was also much persecuted in others. Envious physicians avoided him and denounced him as a cruel person who gloried in cutting into women's bellies. Dr. James Johnson, the respected editor of the *London Medico-Chirurgical Review,* widely circulated in both Great Britain and America, satirized McDowell's ovariectomy, laughing particularly at the rapid recovery of Mrs. Crawford with the words "Credat Judaeus, non ego."[53] In 1827, he had the grace to recant and praise McDowell.

Despite the praise McDowell received from some, he never recovered his standing in his own home town. His practice dwindled because of wild stories people spread about him. The townspeople shunned him socially. The slaves dove into their houses and bolted their doors when he approached. Once he met a huge slave on a solitary strip of road. The man fled but fell on his knees, shrilly praying, after McDowell ordered him to halt. When McDowell quieted him and asked him why he was so afraid, the man answered, "My master...say Dr. McDowell am next to the devil; Dr. McDowell goes around cutting people open and killing them."[54]

McDowell's reputation also suffered because he scorned the pompous tricks of his fellow-doctors. He did not frown while examining patients, or use medical jargon they could not understand, or prescribe all kinds of curatives. He often allowed Nature to heal the sick. So he did not seem to be a competent physician.

A nephew of McDowell also worked against his uncle when McDowell's daughter would have nothing to do with him. He started rumors that the doctor had stolen the credit for the ovariectomy from another man and that he had not even performed the first surgery. Soon this scandal had spread everywhere. McDowell was forced to issue a statement to the contrary accompanied by affidavits from those present at Mrs. Crawford's operation. But Joseph, the nephew, continued his lies.

McDowell quietly continued his life, although his popularity continued to decline and the calumny increased. Once while his wife was ill, people rumored that McDowell had poisoned her in order to marry his apprentice, who, they said, was a woman disguised as a man. McDowell had luckily saved enough during his prosperous years to enable him to buy a plantation where he retired to live the life of a country gentleman. He died at the age of fifty-nine of what was probably acute appendicitis—an ironic end for the man now recognized as the founder of abdominal surgery in America.

MORTON

> "Innovators are rarely received with joy, and established authorities launch into condemnation of newer truths, for...at every crossroads to the future there are a thousand self-appointed guardians of the past."[55]
> Betty MacQuitty

For centuries, physicians and laymen alike considered pain an unavoidable part of life. Had not mankind been condemned to pain in punishment for its disobedience? To ward off pain would be heretical. And so, men like Priestley, Davy, and Hickman, who experimented with gases which could reduce pain, were laughed at and ignored. Besides the religious argument against prevention of pain, fear of gases themselves kept scientists from using inhalants to prevent pain. Scientists noticed that under the influence of gases their patients' pulses slowed, and occasionally these patients became giddy and even unconscious. Advocates of pneumatic medicine were thus pronounced charlatans. Whoever could bring triumph over pain to mankind despite these arguments and the persecution which was sure to follow certainly deserved reward and praise. But this man, William Morton, suffered a lifetime of abuse and libel primarily because of a battle over the questions as to who deserved the credit for discovering anesthesia.

A young doctor, Crawford Long, was perhaps the first to use ether as an inhalant to prevent pain in surgery. He was able to remove tumors from a patient's neck, and he even amputated a young boy's badly damaged finger without pain. But his fellow-doctors complained of his reckless behavior and claimed that he would kill a patient. Superstitious rumors of his devilish practices flew around town. His patients no longer came to him and he was threatened with lynching. And so because of public opinion Long gave up his work with ether. He never realized the importance of his work and never wrote to medical journals to publicize his painless operations. Soon even he forgot about his work with ether.

Another man, however, was busy with his own experiments. William Thomas Green Morton (1819-1868) set up practice as a dentist in 1842. He worked with another dentist, Horace Wells, a bright, enthusiastic, and ambitious young man. Together the men tried to market a new dental solder Wells had invented. This solder was non-corrosive and so did not produce unsightly black lines around the base of the teeth and did not have a bad taste or smell. But they could not attract enough patients to stay in business. Patients did not like the thought of enduring tooth removal and would scuttle down the stairs from the office as quickly as they could. Wells was an impetuous and impatient man. He dissolved his partnership with Morton and went back to his home-town. He was not one to struggle with any enterprise if he did not meet immediate success. Morton's tenacity, on the other hand, enabled him to continue his work.

Soon he enrolled as a Harvard medical student, at the same time continuing his dental practice. He also began searching for ways to reduce pain. He tried many different agents, even mesmerism. He also worked with Wells, who claimed that nitrous oxide could alleviate pain. But an experiment before leading physicians failed and Wells once again abandoned his projects.

Finally, Morton went to a chemistry professor, Dr. Charles Jackson, for advice. Jackson recommended his toothache drops, which were pure ether. Morton found that applying the drops to the tooth did reduce the pain. He then wondered if the whole system could not be influenced by the ether so that its effect would be strengthened and extended. Unlike Jackson, he realized the potential of ether. Over the next years he experimented with various means of administering the substance on animals, but had difficulties with his procedures. He avoided seeking more help from Jackson because he realized that the professor was rather unscrupulous. Jackson had a tremendous obsession with his own power and importance. For seven years he had claimed that he, not Samuel Morse, had invented the telegraph, even taking the issue to the highest courts. And then he claimed that he, not Schonbein, had invented gun-cotton. Morton was afraid that Jackson might guess at the purpose of his experiments and forestall him. But Morton also knew he needed Jackson's advice once more. In discussing his experiments with the chemist, Morton suddenly saw that the ether he had been using for his second round of experiments was not pure.

As soon as he realized that he needed to use pure ether he was able to extract a tooth painlessly from a patient. The very next day he applied for a patent to his secret preparation. He returned to Jackson for a testimonial to support his new product but the chemist would not give one to him. Instead Jackson began spreading rumors about the danger of Morton's preparation. Because Morton was still perfecting his procedures, he had occasional problems with his patients. So he again left his practice to develop an inhaler.

Fortunately, a young doctor, H. J. Bigelow, observed his work and carried his ideas to a prominent physician, John Collins Warren, at the Massachusetts General Hospital. This was the same doctor whom Wells had so disastrously attempted to persuade to use nitrous oxide. Morton was able to remove a patient's tumor without a cry or groan from the patient. Warren was impressed with the demonstration and supported Morton's work.

Thereafter Morton again looked into patenting his discovery. But R. H. Eddy, the Commissioner of Patents, was a close friend of Jackson. He let Jackson know that Morton could make a great deal of money. Immediately Jackson demanded $500 and ten percent of the patent. Morton was astonished at his demand. Although the chemist had given him some technical advice, he was not at all connected with the discovery. But after much argument, Morton gave in to the demand.

Morton then went on with the work of helping others to

benefit from his innovation. He asked Warren for a list of hospitals and charitable trusts so that he could grant them free licenses to use his preparation, the contents of which were still unknown to the medical circle because he added aromatics to disguise ether's characteristic odor. But then the Massachusetts Medical Society objected to their having to pay Morton to use his procedure when hospitals paid nothing. Medical ethics called for all discoverers to make their innovations available at no cost to the world. The physicians banded together and passed a resolution that no one was to use Morton's procedure until he disclosed the contents of the preparation. At the very time Morton was told of this resolution, Warren was preparing to amputate the leg of a young woman. Without the pain-killing substance, she would suffer greatly. Thus, Morton was faced with a difficult decision. He had sacrificed years of hard work, worry, and expense to perfect his procedure and would now be allowed no compensation. He was also afraid of divulging the contents of his preparation when it could be mishandled and the whole idea of killing pain discredited. But Morton was also afraid for the young woman who would suffer needlessly without his discovery. Thinking of her, he announced that the agent he used was ether.

    Although Morton had now done his utmost to help advance medicine in one important area, he was attacked from all sides by envious dentists who spread lies about his procedure and by doctors outside Massachusetts who were left behind their fellow-doctors in Boston. Even European physicians scorned the doctors who were afraid of inflicting pain. Then the religious leaders joined the fray, thundering against ether from their pulpits. But those doctors who realized the value of his contribution hailed Morton's innovation as the greatest discovery of the century. They even talked of the reward Morton should receive.

    Jackson watched the gradual change of opinion. And, as he had before, he began to exaggerate his part in the discovery until he became the inventor and Morton, the bungling, uneducated, and overambitious dentist who had stolen his idea. Over the following years, he sent letters to the French Academy of Sciences, to newspapers, to leading scientists and intellectuals, even to the American Academy—claiming that he, not Morton, had discovered anesthesia (the name given ether by Oliver Wendell Holmes). Morton was devastated by Jackson's deceit. But when he approached Jackson with demands that he issue immediate disclaimers, the chemist cunningly gave Morton his word and then promptly broke it.

The next blow came to Morton when the government began using his treatment, without license or permission, to treat the wounded in the Mexican War. Morton had offered them his treatment a month earlier and they had rejected his discovery, and now they were, in effect, appropriating his patent. Jackson, seeing that Morton's patent was null and void, now announced that he was unwilling to receive the ten percent of the profits he had first requested because he knew the money "would burn in (my) pockets as so much blood money."[56] By this time he hated Morton with what some psychologists have called a psychopathic hatred. He had someone copy all of the dentist's patient records and accounts. Bills were sent to all patients, whether they had paid their debts or not. And action was then taken against them in the circuit courts. Morton arrived at his office to find the waiting room crowded with, on the one hand, indignant, rude patients and, on the other hand, pleading, tearful patients who feared the loss of their property. When the doctor finally figured out what had happened and tried to explain it to his patients, none would believe him. They left him and went to rival dentists. Soon Morton's assistants also left. Now that his livelihood was gone, his creditors descended upon him.

While he was desperately trying to pay off his debts, another claimant to the discovery of anesthesia stepped forward as soon as bills were introduced into Congress to award $100,000 to the discoverer of anesthesia. Horace Wells, hearing this news, claimed that he had discovered the principle of inhalant anesthesia and he had been the first to use nitrous oxide, but not ether. Physicians in authority were appalled at the bitter war being waged over the credit for discovering anesthesia. They were even more appalled when Crawford Long suddenly jumped into the arena. They now had four doctors, all claiming the credit for discovering anesthesia. An official investigation was conducted which dismissed Long's and Wells' claims. Jackson refused to appear before the committee because, he said, he questioned their competence to decide the matter. In the end, Morton was declared the legitimate claimant.

But this investigation did nothing to obviate Jackson's fury or Morton's troubles. Morton's health broke under the constant strain of gossip, intrigues, and poverty. In 1850 the French Academy awarded the Montyon Prize to both Jackson and Morton. Morton was outraged and refused to accept his share of the money, whereupon Jackson stated that he alone had been awarded the prize. When Morton finally agreed to accept a gold medal cast especially for him instead of the money, Jackson claimed that the medal was false.

Over the following years, Congress met several times to decide the issue of the reward of $100,000 and the patent. But each time Morton's hopes were destroyed. After these last rebuffs Morton decided to rebuild his life. He started farming on an acreage he called Etherton. There he won many prizes for his livestock. But when he was appointed Commissioner for the National Agricultural Society and chosen to be delegate to the French Industrial Exhibition, his opponents once more spread scandalous rumors which forced him to abandon his trip. This time the campaign of hate was so terrible that an effigy of him was burned in front of his house before his wife and children.

His troubles seemed over for a while when he was drafted into the army as an anesthetist. For the first time in many years he found comfort in working with his discovery. He was able to buy back his medal which he had pawned for needed money. But his health was poor. He frequently suffered nervous attacks that were certainly the result of twenty years of steady harassment.

In 1868 he read an article that resurrected Jackson's claims and included many of the old libels. Morton traveled to New York to refute the lies. There he suffered a severe attack which led to his death. Some grateful Boston citizens erected a magnificent monument as his tombstone, inscribed with words which credited him with allowing science to control pain.

Jackson came to this monument after five more years of vilifying Morton's name. He had turned to drinking for relief and was by this time an alcoholic. It is said he was drunk when he approached the monument. After reading the inscription, he began to scream. His insanity became clear to all. He was placed in an asylum where he died seven years later, never regaining his senses.

PARACELSUS

"I pleased nobody except the people I cured."[57]
Paracelsus

Many medical forerunnners denounced in their own age have been accepted, even praised, years after their death. However, one innovator, Paracelsus, born in 1493, remains a controversial figure today. Some consider him ridiculous; others say he has received more space than he deserves; one historian calls his books "half-baked and incoherent tomes."[58] And yet others call this heretic "a ferment without which there would be no life."[59] Scholars even founded a Swiss Paracelsus Society in 1942 to restudy his ideas. He incites controversy today as he did in his own day.

As Paracelsus (1493-1541) studied medicine in Italy he began to question what seemed the artificial theories of the ancients upheld in his day. He had observed illnesses long enough to know that experience contradicted the teachings of the ancients. Experience, then, would be his teacher. He decided that he must learn first-hand about healing. Traveling widely through Europe, he learned about illnesses and their remedies from peasants, old wives, craftsmen, and the barber-surgeons. Various specific illnesses he studied were a disease characteristic of miners, fibroid phthisis, and syphilis, a relatively new and little understood disease. He also wrote treatises on mental diseases and kidney and liver disorders. The remedies he learned about and recommended were simple dressings allowing Nature to heal the wound instead of the usual complicated and costly ointments.

He also furthered pharmacology by introducing laudanum, mercury, sulphur, and lead. And he was the first to discuss some new remedies, such as antimony, gold, potassium sulfate, and arsenic. As a result of these and other accomplishments, Paracelsus became well-known among the laity for his seemingly miraculous cures.

But he was poorly received by his fellow-physicians and teachers. When Paracelsus was invited to teach at the University of Basel, he soon antagonized fellow-professors because he continually and belligerently attacked the very basis of all their beliefs. Once he introduced a course of lectures by burning Galen's works and announcing, "My shoe buckles are more learned than Galen,...and my beard knows more than any ancient writer."[60] The combination of these beliefs and his antagonistic and overbearing personality soon alienated all. Classes that had been well-attended because of his innovative thinking—diagnosis of illness from pulse rate and urine analysis, for example—soon were empty. Students did not wish to ally themselves with this unpopular thinker.

Finally his enemies set a trap that would lead to his expulsion. He was asked to treat a wealthy man whom he successfully cured. When the man refused to pay his fee, Paracelsus took him to court. The judge unexpectedly ruled against Paracelsus and then publicly denounced him. His pride thus attacked, Paracelsus left Basel.

Over the next decade, Paracelsus wandered throughout Europe. He constantly sought cures and taught his ideas, always fighting those "old and obstinate dogs who will learn nothing new and are ashamed to recognize their folly."[61] But he was forbidden to teach formally in a university. So he tried to teach through writing. But he soon found that no one would publish his writing. Only in Nuremberg did he find people willing to print his books. But after two works on syphilis appeared, the Leipzig medical faculty protested his writing and prohibited its further publication. After thirteen years of wandering, Paracelsus returned to Salzburg where he died at the age of forty-eight, leaving most of his possessions to the poor except for his manuscripts which he gave to a barber-surgeon, not trusting them in the hands of a learned doctor.

Fortunately some of these manuscripts remain, although much of the writing is mystical and difficult to evaluate. But his ideas are noteworthy. The practice of medicine, he says, is based on four principles. First, the physician must observe and know nature to understand life. Second, he must understand astronomy, for as the stars are governed by law so is man governed by environment. Third, he must study chemistry to understand how the body lives. Fourth, he must practice virtue—devotion to his patient and to his professional ethics. Paracelsus also believed that in man an active force, or *archaeus,* provided life, and that disease was a weakening of this vital force. These and other ideas mystically expressed have clouded his philosophy of medicine, making it difficult to judge as a contribution to medicine.

Clearly his greatest contribution was his revolt against ancient medicine in a day when the rebel was struck down. Paracelsus called for a new medicine based on experience, not ancient authority: "he opened a path for men with bold ideas to follow."[62]

PASTEUR

"If I have at times disturbed the calm of your academies by discussions of too great an intensity, it is only because I wanted to defend the cause of truth."[63]
Louis Pasteur

When Louis Pasteur (1822-1895) graduated from college with his Bachelor of Science degree in 1842, he received a "mediocre" in chemistry. And yet he became an accomplished chemist and microbiologist. During his lifetime he discovered a new class of isomeric substances when he proved that racemic acid contained two types of crystals that together polarized light neither to the left nor to the right. He was the first to produce and use vaccines for anthrax, rabies, and chicken cholera. He helped to disprove the theory of spontaneous generation when he advanced the germ theory. He even saved the wine, beer, and silk industries through this new theory. But these accomplishments were not immediately accepted. He met with constant opposition from doctors and fellow-scientists.

Pasteur's experiments disproving spontaneous generation and proving the germ theory caused great scientific uproar. The beer and wine industries were having many problems with diseases that ruined their products. Pasteur began his work by examining the yeasts of beer and found differences between the yeast globules of sound beer and those of sour beer. After more research he concluded that microorganisms cause fermentation and that failure of fermentation resulted either from the organisms' absence or from their inability to grow properly. After many detailed experiments that included air filtration and the exposure of liquids to mountain air, he concluded that the organisms were not spontaneously generated, but rather came from similar organisms in the air. He suggested sterilization of wine and beer through a heating process later called pasteurization and generalized to include other food products like milk.

Pasteur read a paper describing his experiments and his conclusions to the Academy of Medicine. The result was indignant anger; how could this lay person who was not even a doctor dispute the doctrine of spontaneous generation? Pasteur's responses to his opponents were always hot-headed and impetuous. So when he answered them with angry charges of his own, he was ejected from the meeting and later even challenged to a duel by one of the doctors.

But this antagonism did not stop Pasteur from continuing related research in another industry. The silkworm industry was almost devastated in France when a disease began attacking the silkworm eggs. Pasteur accepted the challenge of preventing this disease although he was unfamiliar with silkworms. In three years he isolated the bacilli of the two silkworm diseases and found a method for preventing disease as well as for detecting diseased silkworms. But in so doing, he angered those who were unwilling to change traditional methods of raising silkworms. He probably also angered them with his zealous attacks on their methods. Some of the dealers even spread rumors about Pasteur that eventually reached the newspapers. Pasteur's father-in-law discussed one of the rumors in a letter to his daughter, saying that he had heard that Pasteur's process had failed and that he had had to flee from the village where he was staying while pursuers threw stones at him.

But difficulties like these did not cause Pasteur to give up his work in discouragement, although his health did begin to deteriorate. In 1868, he suffered a stroke that left him partially paralyzed; however, he was able to return to his work with the fatal cattle disease, anthrax. Within two years he isolated the bacterium that caused the disease and then developed a vaccine. This time he provoked Robert Koch, a German physician who was doing much of the same research, although Koch had not developed a vaccine. Koch and his assistants vehemently opposed Pasteur and his methods because they did not consider him qualified to study diseases; he was, by training, merely a chemist, they said. When Pasteur invited Koch to an exchange of ideas, Koch refused, instead publishing a paper denouncing much of Pasteur's work.

Perhaps the greatest conflict surrounded Pasteur's last major contribution—the development of a rabies inoculation. Pasteur successfully inoculated a young boy who had been bitten by a rabid dog and then he began to inoculate others. Sometimes the treatments were not successful and patients died. Doctors waiting for just this result condemned him as an assassin. Political and medical journals campaigned against him. Physicians and students split into factions for and against him. The strain of constant argument caused him to travel to the Riviera for rest because of signs of heart disease. Fortunately, some prominent physicians and professors interceded for him, and the controversy abated. His discovery was gradually accepted as its success became apparent. And with the acceptance came a large endowment that allowed him to establish the Institute Pasteur in Paris, a research institute that Pasteur directed until his death in 1895.

Pasteur's life was a curious mixture of tremendous medical discoveries and advancements and yet violent conflicts with those who held to the established doctrines of his day. Pasteur was eventually honored and respected for his work, but not until he overcame much opposition. He just never allowed obstacles to stop his work; "rather, he ran down and over orthodoxy like a roaring cavalry charge"[64] fighting passionately for truth.

SERVETUS

> "...for no great discovery has ever been immediately accepted. Rather, in medicine it seems that the reverse is true, and everyone must go through a period of trial and even censure before what seems the obvious truth is recognized generally... But such slow acceptance prevents the real discoveries from being known and widely accepted earlier, and many lives are thus sacrificed needlessly."[65]
>
> Frank Slaughter

Miguel Serveto or Servetus (c.1510-1553), was born in the early 1500's in Spain. Since he was interested in various fields of thought, he studied theology, law, and medicine. To study medicine he traveled to Paris so that he might work with various professors, one of which, Jacobus Sylvius, occasionally dissected a human body, which was very unusual because dissection had been banned by the church. In studying the heart, Servetus could find none of the pores that Galen had said existed in the dividing wall of the heart and allowed blood to flow from one ventricle directly into the other. After further study he recorded his own theory:

> This connection is not made across the wall of the heart, but very cunningly: the blood is pumped out of the right ventricle and conducted to the lungs. The lungs make the blood bright and fresh, and then, via the arteries it is passed to the veins, from which it is pumped into the left ventricle and so reaches all the arteries in the body.[66]

Servetus had discovered pulmonary circulation and hinted at systematic circulation.

However, his interest in medicine was superseded by that of theology, for him an unfortunate interest. He wished to reform the church and to change its unenlightened beliefs. In his *Christianismi Restitutione,* published in France in 1553, he outlined what he considered the errors of the church. He also discussed Galen's errors. He consequently aroused the enmity of both religious and scientific leaders. First, he was questioning church doctrine. Second, he was studying the human body when dissection had been banned by Pope Boniface VIII. Third, he was questioning the long-accepted medical authority, Galen.

But he did not stop here. He sent a copy of his book to the Protestant reformer Calvin, hoping to discuss his ideas with him. Calvin accepted neither Servetus nor his thinking, calling him a "limb of Satan" and warning him never to set foot in Geneva at the risk of his life. Ironically enough, Calvin then denounced Servetus to the Catholic Inquisition, sending them whatever condemning information, even personal correspondence, he could find.

As a result, Servetus was arrested, although he was able to escape to a monastery where he hid for three months. Then in July, 1553, he foolhardily journeyed to Geneva where he was recognized. Calvin had Servetus imprisoned and tortured for three months, meanwhile allowing him no defense at his trial. On October 27, 1553, he was condemned to be burned at the stake. He begged to be executed by the sword, but instead, Calvin ordered Servetus to be slowly burned to death—in damp straw.

Servetus' great "error" had been to question church doctrine, but he had further condemned himself by questioning indisputable medical doctrine set forth by Galen in 150 A.D., 1300 years earlier.

POSTSCRIPT

You and I do not know what the future will bring. But, from the perspective of history we can understand the enormous tensions that are as old as the world and as timely as the headlines of today. The inevitable battles in each generation between the past and the future, between those who talk about change, those whose leadership makes change happen and those who worry about and resist change are struggles to be expected and accepted. Hopefully, *Medical Mavericks, Volume I* helps us to see beyond the passing moment to realize that the task of each generation is to blaze trails and to build roads and highways for the next and to inspire anew those whose achievements and ideals are yet to become history.

CHRONOLOGICAL LIST

Hippocrates	460 B.C.
Claudius Galenus	130 A.D.
Roger Bacon	1220-1292
Pietro d'Abano	1250-1315
Paracelsus	1493-1541
Miguel Serveto or Servetus	1510-1553
William Harvey	1578-1657
Zabdiel Boylston	1680-1766
Leopold Auenbrugger	1722-1809
Antoine Lavoisier	1743-1794
Ephraim McDowell	1771-1830
Henry Hill Hickman	1800-1830
William Morton	1819-1868
Elizabeth Blackwell	1821-1910
Louis Pasteur	1822-1895
Joseph Lister	1827-1912
Georg Groddeck	1866-1934
Joseph Goldberger	1874-1929

FOOTNOTES

1. Leopold Auenbrugger quoted by James Joseph Walsh, Makers of Modern Medicine (rpt. 1907; New York: Books for Libraries Press, 1970), pp. 67-68.
2. Review quoted by Walsh, pp. 71-72.
3. Henry Thomas Schnittkind, Living Biographies of Great Scientists, (Henry Thomas and Dana Lee Thomas, pseuds.) Garden City, N. Y.: Garden City Books, 1959, p. 15.
4. Schnittkind, p. 17.
5. Schnittkind, p. 20.
6. Gerhard Venzmer, Five Thousand Years of Medicine, trans. Marion Koenig (New York, Taplinger, 1968), p. 155.
7. Elizabeth Blackwell quoted in 400 Years of a Doctor's life, ed. George Rosen and Beate Caspari-Rosen (New York: Schuman, 1947), pp. 182-183.
8. Elizabeth Blackwell quoted in Geoffrey Marks and William K. Beatty, Women in White (New York: Charles Scribner's Sons, 1972), pp. 84-87.
9. Charles A. Lee quoted in Elizabeth Blackwell, Pioneer Work in Opening the Medical Profession to Women (rpt. 1895; New York: Schocken Books, 1977), pp. 64-65.
10. Dr. Stephen Smith, speech, Jan. 25, 1911 in New York City, quoted in Esther Lovejoy, Women Doctors of the World (New York: Macmillan, 1957), p. 47.
11. Dr. Stephen Smith quoted in Marks and Beatty, pp. 87-88.
12. Marks and Beatty, pp. 87-88.
13. Blackwell, p. 190.
14. Bruce Barton quoted in The New Dictionary of Thoughts, comp. Tyrone Edwards (New York: Doubleday, 1955), p. 447.
15. J. Kilpatrick quoted in John T. Barrett, "The Inoculation

Controversy in Puritan New England," <u>Bulletin of the History of Medicine</u>, 12 (1942), p. 174.
16. Logan Clendening, <u>The Romance of Medicine</u>, (Garden City, N. Y.: Garden City Publishing Co., 1933), p. 213.
17. Barrett, pp. 174-175.
18. James Thacher, <u>American Medical Biography</u> (rpt. 1828; New York: Milford House, 1967), pp. 188-189.
19. Pietro d'Abano quoted in Lynn Thorndike, "Peter of Abano: A Medieval Scientist." In <u>Annual Report for the Year 1919</u> (Washington, D. C.: American Historical Association, 1923), pp. 321-322.
20. Pietro d'Abano quoted in Thorndike, p. 322.
21. Thomas of Strasbourg quoted in Thorndike, p. 323.
22. Savonarola quoted in Thorndike, p. 324.
23. Savonarola quoted in Thorndike, pp. 324-5.
24. Sir Thomas Clifford Allbutt, <u>Greek Medicine in Rome: the Fitzpatrick Lectures on the History of Medicine Delivered at the Royal College of Physicians of London in 1909-1910</u> (rpt. 1921; New York: Benjamin Blom, 1970), p. 295.
25. Galen quoted in Tibor Doby, <u>Discoverers of Blood Circulation, from Aristotle to the Times of daVinci and Harvey</u> (London: Abelard-Schuman, 1963), p. 50.
26. Joseph Goldberger quoted in Elizabeth W. Etheridge, <u>The Butterfly Caste: the Social History of Pellagra in the South</u> (Westport, Conn.: Greenwood Publ. Co., 1972), pp. 86-87.
27. The United Daughters of the Confederacy, Etheridge, pp. 149-150.
28. Joseph Goldberger quoted in Etheridge, p. 101.
29. Paul de Kruif quoted in Etheridge, p. 186.
30. Joseph Goldberger quoted in Etheridge, p. 186.
31. Joseph Goldberger quoted in Etheridge, pp. 220-221.
32. Georg Groddeck, presentation to the Psychoanalytic Congress at the Hague, 1920.
33. Georg Groddeck, letter to Sigmund Freud, May 27,

1917, quoted in Carl M. Grossman and Sylvia Grossman, The Wild Analyst: the Life and Work of Georg Groddeck (New York: Columbia University Press, 1954), pp. 66-69.
34. Sigmund Freud, letter to Georg Groddeck, quoted in Alan Watts, "The Mystic More Freudian than Freud," New Republic, 152: 22-4, May 1, 1965.
35. Groddeck in The Psychic Origin and Psychoanalytical Treatment of Organic Disease, quoted in Grossman, pp. 80-81.
36. Groddeck, The Book of the It, quoted in Martin Grotjahn, Georg Groddeck 1866-1934, the Untamed Analyst," Psychoanalytic Pioneers, ed. Franz Alexander et al. (New York: Basic Books, 1966), pp. 312-314.
37. William Harvey quoted in "Scientific Papers," The Harvard Classics, 38 (New York: P. S. Collier & Son, 1910), pp .76-77.
38. Arturo Castiglioni, A History of Medicine, trans. and ed. E. D. Krumbhaar (New York: Knopf, 1947), pp. 519-520.
39. Ralph Herman Major, A History of Medicine (Springfield, IL: Charles C. Thomas, 1954), I, pp. 496-497.
40. Sir William Hale-White, Great Doctors of the Nineteenth Century (rpt. 1935; Freeport, N. Y.: Books for Libraries Press, 1970), p. 153.
41. Hale-White, p. 23.
42. Rene Fulop-Miller, Triumph over Pain, trans. Eden and Cedar Paul (New York: Lieberary Guild of America, 1938), pp. 82-86.
43. Sir James Elliott, Outlines of Greek and Roman Medicine (rpt. 1914; Boston: Longwood Press, 1978), pp. 51-52.
44. Hippocrates quoted in Elliott, p. 28.
45. Coffinhal quoted in Kenneth Walker, The Story of Medicine (New York: Oxford University Press, 1954), pp. 155-156.

46. Henry Thomas Schnittkind, Living Biographies of Great Scientists (Henry Thomas and Dana Lee Thomas, pseudonyms) Garden City, N. Y.: Garden City Books, 1959, p. 76.
47. Schnittkind, pp. 76-77.
48. Sir James Young Simpson quoted in M. E. M. Walker, Pioneers of Public Health: the Story of Some Benefactors of the Human Race (rpt. 1930; Freeport, N. Y.: Books for Libraries Press, 1968), p. 154.
49. The editor of The Lancet, quoted in Richard B. Fisher, Joseph Lister, 1827-1912 (New York: Stein and Day, 1977), p. 164.
50. The Lancet, quoted in A. J. Youngson, The Scientific Revolution in Victorian Medicine (New York: Holmes & Meier Publ., 1979), pp. 207-8.
51. Professor Tyndale quoted in Theodore Cianfrani. A Short History of Obstetrics and Gynecology (Springfield, Ill.: Charles C. Thomas, 1960), pp. 282-283.
52. Ephraim McDowell in letter to Dr. James, Sept., 1819 quoted in James Thomas Flexner, Doctors on Horseback: Pioneers of American Medicine (New York: Viking, 1937), pp. 149-150.
53. Dr. James Johnson quoted in Frank Jirka, American Doctors of Destiny (Freeport, N. Y.: Books for Libraries Press, 1970), pp. 77-78.
54. Flexner, pp. 151-152.
55. Betty MacQuitty, Victory over Pain: Morton's Discovery of Anaesthesia (New York: Taplinger Pub. Co., pp. 102-103.
56. Charles Jackson quoted by MacQuitty, pp. 131-132.
57. Paracelsus quoted in John Michael Francis Camp, The Healter's Art (New York: Taplinger, 1977), pp. 73-74.
58. Ralph Herman Major, A History of Medicine (Springfield, Ill.: Charles C. Thomas, 1954), I, p. 392.
59. Major, p. 392
60. Paracelsus quoted in Camp, pp. 73-74.

61. Paracelsus quoted in Sarah Regal Reidman, <u>Masters of the Scalpel</u> (Chicago: Rand MacNally, 1962), p. 54.
62. Felix Marti-Ibanez, <u>The Crystal Arrow</u> (New York: C. N. Potter, 1964), p. 532.
63. Louis Pasteur quoted in Rene Jules Dubos, <u>Louis Pasteur, Free Lance of Science</u> (Boston: Little Brown, 1950), p. 76.
64. Wayne Martin, <u>Medical Heroes and Heretics</u> (Old Greenwich, Conn.: Devin-Adair, 1977), p. 3.
65. Frank Slaughter, <u>Immortal Magyar: Semmelweis, Conqueror of Childbed Fever</u> (New York: Schuman, 1950), p. 74.
66. Gerhard Venzmer, <u>Five Thousand Years of Medicine</u>, trans. Marion Koenig (New York: Taplinger, 1968), pp. 168-169.

BIBLIOGRAPHY

Allbutt, Sir Thomas Clifford. <u>Greek Medicine in Rome: The Fitzpatrick Lectures on the History of Medicine Delivered at the Royal College of Physicians of London in 1909-1910</u>. Rpt. 1921; New York: Benjamin Blom, 1970.

Barrett, John T. "The Inoculation Controversy in Puritan New England," <u>Bulletin of the History of Medicine</u>, 12 (1942), pp. 169-188.

Blackwell, Elizabeth. <u>Pioneer Work in Opening the Medical Profession to Women</u>. Rpt. 1895; New York: Schocken Books, 1977.

Camp, John Michael Francis. <u>The Healer's Art</u>. New York: Taplinger, 1977.

Castiglioni, Arturo. <u>A History of Medicine</u>. Trans. and ed. E. D. Krumbhaar. New York: Knopf, 1947.

Chauvois, Louis. <u>William Harvey</u>. New York: Philosophical Library, 1957.

Cianfrani, Theodore. <u>A Short History of Obstetrics and Gynecology</u>. Springfield, Ill.: Charles C. Thomas, 1960.

Clendening, Logan. <u>The Romance of Medicine</u>. Garden City, N. Y.: Garden City Publishing Co., 1933.

Debus, Alan G. <u>The English Paracelsians</u>. New York: Watts, 1965.

Doby, Tibor. <u>Discoverers of Blood Circulation</u>. London: Abelard-Schuman, 1963.

Dolan, John Patrick and William N. Adam-Smith. *Health and Society*. New York: Seabury Press, 1978.

Dubos, Rene Jules. *Louis Pasteur, Free Lance of Science*. Boston: Little Brown, 1950.

Duffy, John. *The Healers: The Rise of the Medical Establishment*. New York: McGraw, 1976.

Elliott, Sir James. *Outlines of Greek and Roman Medicine*. Rpt. 1914; Boston: Longwood Press, 1978.

Etheridge, Elizabeth W. *The Butterfly Caste: The Social History of Pellagra in the South*. Westport, Conn.: Greenwood Publ. Co., 1972. In *Contributions in American History*, No. 17.

Fisher, Richard B. *Joseph Lister, 1827-1912*. New York: Stein and Day, 1977.

Flexner, James Thomas. *Doctors on Horseback: Pioneers of American Medicine*. New York: Viking, 1937.

400 Years of a Doctor's Life. Ed. George Rosen and Beate Caspari-Rosen. New York: Schuman, 1947.

Freeman, Walter. *The Psychiatrist, Personalities and Patterns*. New York: Grune & Stratton, 1968.

Fuer, Lewis Samuel. *The Scientific Intellectual*. New York: Basic Books, 1963.

Fulop-Miller, Rene. *Triumph over Pain*. Trans. Eden and Cedar Paul. New York: Literary Guild of America, 1938.

Garland, Joseph. The Story of Medicine. Boston: Houghton Mifflin, 1949.

Glasscheib, Hermann Samuel. The March of Medicine: The Emergence and Triumph of Modern Medicine. Trans. Mervyn Savill. New York: Putnam, 1964.

Grossman, Carl M. and Sylvia Grossman. The Wild Analyst; the Life and Work of Georg Groddeck. New York: George Braziller, 1965.

Grotjahn, Martin. "Georg Groddeck, 1866-1934, the Untamed Analyst." In Psychoanalytic Pioneers Ed. Franz Alexander, Samuel Eisenstien and Martin Grotjahn. New York: Basic Books, 1966.

Haggard, Howard Wilcox. The Doctor in History. New Haven: Yale University Press, 1934.

Haggard, Howard Wilcox. Mystery, Magic, and Medicine: The Rise of Medicine from Superstition to Science. Garden City, N. Y.: Doubleday, Doran & Co., 1933.

Hale-White, Sir William. Great Doctors of the Nineteenth Century. Rpt. 1935; Freeport, N. Y.: Books for Libraries Press, 1970.

Hannaway, Owen. "Lavoisier," In The McGraw-Hill Encyclopedia of World Biography. New York: McGraw-Hill Book Co., 1973.

Harvey, William. "Scientific Papers," The Harvard Classics, 38. New York: P. S. Collier & Son, 1910.

Hathaway, Esse Virginia. Partners in Progress. Rpt. 1935; Freeport, N. Y.: Books for Libraries Press, 1968.

Jirka, Frank. American Doctors of Destiny. Rpt. 1940; Freeport, N. Y.: Books for Libraries Press, 1970.

Lambert, Samuel Waldron and George M. Goodwin. Medical Leaders from Hippocrates to Osler. Indianapolis: The Bobbs-Merrill Co., 1929.

Lovejoy, Esther. Women Doctors of the World. New York: Macmillan, 1957.

Ludovici, Laurence James. The Discovery of Anaesthesia. New York: Crowell, 1962.

Lyons, Albert S. and R. Joseph Petrucelli, II. Medicine: An Illustrated History. New York: Harry N. Abrams, Inc., 1978.

MacQuitty, Betty. Victory over Pain; Morton's Discovery of Anaesthesia. New York: Taplinger Publ. Co., 1971.

Major, Ralph Herman. A History of Medicine. Springfield, Il.: Charles C. Thomas, 1954.

Marks, Geoffrey and William K. Beatty. Women in White. New York: Charles Scribner's Sons, 1972.

Marti-Ibanez, Felix, The Crystal Arrow. New York: C. N. Potter, 1964.

Martin, Wayne. Medical Heroes and Heretics. Old Greenwich, Conn.: Devin-Adair, 1977.

Metchnikoff, Elie. The Founders of Modern Medicine: Pasteur, Koch, Lister. Rpt. 1939; Freeport, N. Y.: Books for Libraries Press, 1971.

Montgomery, Elizabeth Rider. The Story Behind Great Medical Discoveries. New York: Dodd, Mead, 1945.

Osler, Sir William. The Evolution of Modern Medicine. New Haven: Yale University Press, 1923.

Phillips, Eustace Dockray. Aspects of Greek Medicine. New York: St. Martin's Press, 1973.

Reidman, Sarah Regal. Masters of the Scalpel: the Story of Surgery. Chicago: Rand MacNally, 1962.

Rolleston, Sir Humphrey. "The Reception of Harvey's Doctrine of the Circulation of the Blood in England as Exhibited in the Writings of Two Contemporaries." In Essays on the History of Medicine. Ed. Charles Singer and Henry E. Sigerist. Rpt. 1924; Books for Libraries Press, 1968.

Schnittkind, Henry Thomas. Living Biographies of Great Scientists. (Henry Thomas and Dana Lee Thomas, pseudonyms) Garden City, N.Y.: Garden City Books, 1959.

Shaftel, Norman. "The Evolution of American Medical Literature." In History of American Medicine: A Symposium. Ed. Felix Marti-Ibanez. New York: MD Publications, 1958., No. 5, pp. 95-118.

Sigerist, Henry Ernst. The Great Doctors: A Biographical History of Medicine. Trans. Eden and Cedar Paul. New York: Norton, 1933.

Singer, Charles Joseph. A Short History of Medicine. Rpt. 1928; New York: Oxford University Press, 1962.

Slaughter, Frank. Immortal Magyar: Semmelweis, Conqueror of Childbed Fever. New York: Schuman, 1950.

Thacher, James. American Medical Biography. Rpt. 1828; New York: Milford House, 1967.

Thorndike, Lynn. "Peter of Abano: A Medieval Scientist." In Annual Report for the Year 1919. Washington, D. C.: American Historical Association, 1923, Vol. I, pp. 315-326.

Venzmer, Gerhard. Five Thousand Years of Medicine. Trans. Marion Koenig. New York: Taplinger, 1968.

Walker, Kenneth. The Story of Medicine. New York: Oxford University Press, 1954.

Walker, M. E. M. Pioneers of Public Health: The Story of Some Benefactors of the Human Race. Rpt. 1930; Freeport, N. Y.: Books for Libraries Press, 1968.

Walsh, James Joseph. Makers of Modern Medicine. Rpt. 1907; Freeport, N. Y.: Books for Libraries, 1970.

Watts, Alan. "The Mystic More Freudian than Freud," The New Republic Vol. 152, pp. 22-24, May 1, 1965.

Woglom, William Henry. Discoverers for Medicine. New Haven: Yale University Press, 1949.

Young, Agnes (Brooks). Scalpel, Men Who Made Surgery. (Agatha Young, pseudonym.) New York: Random House, 1956.

Youngson, A. J. The Scientific Revolution in Victorian Medicine. New York: Holmes and Meier Pub., 1979.

VOLUME II

What lies ahead in Volume II? What compelling vignettes will it contain?

A great deal of material has already been collected, reviewed and written. But, the final drafts have not yet been formalized. There is still time for you to send me your ideas. Let me know who you would like to read about. They can be famous or infamous just so they changed medical history.

Your input will be appreciated and help me to write an even better second volume.

Just send your valued comments to:

Hugh D. Riordan, M.D.
The Center
3100 N. Hillside Avenue
Wichita, Kansas 67219 USA

ABOUT THE PUBLISHER

Bio-Communications Press is a service of the Olive W. Garvey Center for the Improvement of Human Functioning, Inc. The Center is a non-profit medical, research and educational organization funded through grants from corporations and foundations and contributions from individuals.

The Center has established three major divisions to carry out its mission of seeking to help stimulate an epidemic of health. These are the ABNA Clinical Research Center, The Bio-Communications Research Institute and The Biomedical Synergistics Education Institute.

To learn more about The Center just send your note of request together with a stamped self-addressed #10 envelope to:

The Center
3100 N. Hillside Avenue
Wichita, Kansas 67219 USA

Bio-Communications Press

THERE'S MORE

Bio-Communications Press fulfills a unique niche by publishing fascinating books for select audiences. These books are written by skilled professionals who have demonstrated both a profound interest in their subject matter and the capacity to clearly communicate that interest in an understandable way.

Although our books are not for everyone, we believe what we publish makes a valuable addition to the personal library of anyone who appreciates being well informed on the subject matter they contain.

To receive a list of books currently available from Bio-Communications Press or to be among the first to know when a new book is about to be released, just return the coupon today.

Bio-Communications Press, 3100 N. Hillside, Wichita, Kansas 67219 U.S.A.

Please send me information about available books.

NAME _____

ADDRESS _____

CITY _____

STATE _____ ZIP CODE _____

NOTES

NOTES

NOTES

NOTES

NOTES